Recent Results in Cancer Research 147

Springer
Berlin
Heidelberg
New York
Barcelona
Budapest
Hong Kong
London
Milan
Paris
Santa Clara
Singapore
Tokyo

K. J. Oldhafer H. Lang
R. Pichlmayr † (Eds.)

Isolated Liver Perfusion for Hepatic Tumors

With 62 Figures and 25 Tables

Springer

Priv.-Doz. Dr. med. Karl J. Oldhafer
Dr. med. Hauke Lang
Prof. Dr. med. Rudolf Pichlmayr†

Medizinische Hochschule Hannover
Klinik für Abdominal- und Transplantationschirurgie
Konstanty-Gutschow-Straße 8
D-30625 Hannover

ISBN-13:978-3-642-80462-5 e-ISBN-13:978-3-642-80460-1
DOI: 10.1007/978-3-642-80460-1

ISSN 0080-0015

Library of Congress Cataloging-in-Publication Data
Isolated liver perfusion in hepatic tumors / K.J. Oldhafer, H. Lang, R. Pichlmayr (eds.). (Recent results in cancer research, ISSN 0080-0015; 147) Includes bibliographical references and index. ISBN-13:978-3-642-80462-5 1. Liver–Cancer–Chemotherapy–Congresses. 2. Isolation perfusion (Physiology)–Congresses. I. Oldhafer, K.J. (Karl J.), 1960– . II. Lang, H. (Hauke), 1963– . III. Pichlmayr, R. (Rudolf), 1932–1997. IV. Series. [DNLM: 1. Perfusion. 2. Liver–surgery. 3. Liver Neoplasms–therapy. WI 770 I85 1997] RC261.R35 vol. 147 [RC280.L5] 616.99′4 s–dc21 [616.99′436] DNLM/DLC for Library of Congress

Production: PRO EDIT GmbH, D-69126 Heidelberg
Typesetting: K+V Fotosatz GmbH, D-64743 Beerfelden

SPIN 10571841 19/3133-5 4 3 2 1 0 – Printed on acid-free paper

Preface

The contributions in this book were originally presented at the workshop "Research and Clinical Application of Isolated Liver Perfusion for Hepatic Tumors" held on 28 February to 1 March 1997 in Hanover, Germany. The workshop was planned to bring together groups working with isolated liver perfusion techniques worldwide. Experts from various countries were invited to present and discuss their experimental data and clinical results. Groups from Japan, The Netherlands, Sweden and the USA participated. At the beginning, oncologists, surgeons and pathologists presented possible indications and the oncological background for therapeutic isolated liver perfusion from their points of view. Based on data from previous studies about locoregional chemotherapy and based on the pathology of metastasis, it could be concluded that there is a place for isolated liver perfusion in the therapy of liver cancer. Second, different surgical techniques of isolated liver perfusion were presented. These techniques varied from a percutaneous approach with extracorporeal chemofiltration to extended open abdominal surgery. Perfusion of the liver without a considerable amount of drug reaching the systemic circulation proved to be possible. The complex procedure with complicated extracorporeal perfusion technique represented a disadvantage of the methods presented. Further studies should simplify the technical and surgical aspects. Intraoperative and postoperative management of patients undergoing isolated liver perfusion were also discussed. Coagulopathy was one important aspect which can occur during isolated liver perfusion. The percentage of leakage determined systemic side effects. Thus, leakage monitoring could be useful when severely toxic drugs are used (e.g. tumor necrosis factor, TNF). Several chemotherapeutic drugs with potential for isolated liver perfusion were presented. It turned out that mitomycin C could not be recommended due to its severe hepatotoxicity. TNF, however, represents a promising drug for this approach. It acts within 1 h and is very effective in the high concentrations that can be achieved in isolated perfusion. Early clinical results with TNF in isolated liver perfusion were presented and seemed promising. Hyperthermia is also used in isolated liver perfusion as an adjunct to chemotherapy. It was shown that hyperthermia, even alone, can be very effective in tumor cell killing. Hyperthermia can be achieved in liver perfusion by heating the perfusion circuit. Finally, a difficult but important issue is the evaluation of postoperative results. While the primary aim is to produce as much tumor necrosis as possible, it may be difficult to differentiate between vital and necrotic tumor cells. Positron emission tomography scanning was presented as a possible tool.

In the future, isolated liver perfusion may open new fields of therapy. For example, it may be used to deliver liver-specific suicide genes. Further, non-recirculating anoxic liver perfusion has been used after liver resection to treat the remaining liver in terms of adjuvant chemotherapy.

We would like to thank all authors for their support and contributions.

During the preparation of this volume the head of our department, Prof. Dr. Rudolf Pichlmayr, died at the congress of the International Surgical Society in Acapulco, Mexico, Prof. Pichlmayr initiated our program of isolated liver perfusion in Hanover. At the workshop we enjoyed intensive discussions with him and developed new plans for the future. Prof. Pichlmayr was a very important person for the Hanover program of isolated liver perfusion. He stimulated and supported us in all aspects of the establishment of this procedure in the division of Abdominal and Transplantation Surgery of Hanover Medical School. We want to continue this work and to realize the plans we founded with him.

Hanover, April 1998

Karl J. Oldhafer
Hauke Lang

Contents

I. Indication

II. Technique/Anaesthesia

III. High-Dose Chemoperfusion

IV. Tumor Necrosis Factor

V. Radiological Control of Tumor Response

VI. Future Aspects

List of Contributors*

* The address of the principal author is given on the first page of each contribution.

[1] Page on which contribution begins.

I. Indication

Are There Indications for Intraarterial Hepatic Chemotherapy or Isolated Liver Perfusion? The Case of Liver Metastases from Colorectal Cancer

P. Rougier

Service d'hepato-gastroenterologie, Hopital Ambroise Parè,
9, avenue Charles de Gaulle, F-92104 Boulogne cedex, France

Abstract

Intraarterial hepatic chemotherapy (IAHC) has been used for many years to treat liver tumors (primary or secondary) if no extrahepatic extension exists, when no resection is feasible, and when no active systemic chemotherapy is available. Liver metastases from colorectal cancer represent one of the best indications, and many trials have demonstrated that IAHC is an efficient treatment. Some of these trials were randomized and have demonstrated that IAHC significantly increases the response rate using IA FUDR compared to its systemic administration, and increases the overall survival compared to symptomatic treatment or systemic bolus 5FU. Liver toxicity and extrahepatic progression are the two main limiting factors which can be reduced using new protocols and combinations with systemic chemotherapy. New drugs such as THP adriamycin will become available for IAHC in the future. Isolated liver perfusion adds to IAHC an extracorporal extraction and allows the use of higher doses of chemotherapy. Its efficacy has been suggested in small phase II trials; however, its relative complexity and the lack of clear demonstration of its efficacy compared to the most recent and effective systemic chemotherapies used alone or in combination with IAHC prevent the recommendation of its use outside clinical trials. IAHC and isolated liver perfusion are two active locoregional treatments which can be combined with surgical resection and/or systemic chemotherapy and warrant further development, if possible, in randomized trials.

Introduction

Intraarterial hepatic chemotherapy (IAHC) and isolated liver perfusion (ILP) have been developed to treat tumor confined to the liver (i.e., mainly liver metastases from colorectal cancer, hepatocellular carcinomas, neuroendocrine tumors, liver metastases from ocular melanoma, and liver metastases from abdominal leiomyosarcomas). Liver metastases from colorectal cancer comprise the most frequent indication for local treatment. They are confined to

Recent Results in Cancer Research, Vol. 147

the liver in about 15% of cases and are resectable in approximately half of such cases. The prognosis for patients with unresectable tumors is poor, even when the lesions are restricted to the liver. One-year survival ranges from 13% for patients with a performance status (PS) of >0 and an elevated alkaline phosphatase (AP) level to 47% for those with a PS of 0 and normal AP (Rougier et al.. 1995). Locoregional therapies, especially IAHC were developed during the early 1980s when no efficient systemic chemotherapy was available. Since then, the efficacy of IAHC has been demonstrated in many trials (Allen-Mersh et al.. 1994; Chang et al.. 1987; Hohn et al.. 1989; Kemeny et al.. 1987; Martin et al.. 1990; Rougier et al.. 1992) but its value compared with modern systemic chemotherapy has never been fully established (Kemeny 1992; O'Connell 1992; Patt 1993a, b). Nor has there been any interest in combining IAHC with systemic chemotherapy. The therapeutic value of ILP remains to be demonstrated in comparison with IAHC and systemic treatments.

Rationale for the Use of IAHC

Use of IAHC is a logical approach for treating tumors confined to the liver based on anatomical and pharmacokinetic reasons.

1. In contrast to the healthy liver, which is mainly vascularized by the portal vein, liver metastases > 5 mm are irrigated by the hepatic arteries (Breedis and Young 1954).
2. The healthy liver is a major site of detoxification for many drugs. A high extraction rate for drugs infused via the hepatic arterial route allows an important decrease in systemic concentration (Chen and Gross 1980).

These two properties result in increased drug concentration at the tumor level, particularly the fluoropyrimidines. 5-Fluoro-2′-deoxyuridine (FUDR) has a high hepatic clearance, and its concentration in the liver and metastases is higher than that of 5-fluorouracil (5FU Ensminger and Gyves 1983); it is especially higher after hepatic arterial infusion than after portal infusion.

Results of IAHC

Phase II IAHC trials, initially using 5FU with an exteriorized catheter and an external electric pump, produced interesting results, with a 30–80% response rate; unfortunately complications were frequent. Subsequently, the development of totally implantable pumps using FUDR, which required an external refill only every 2 weeks, made IAHC more feasible. This system produced encouraging results in many phase II trials, with a 40–50% response rate and 10–20% complete responses, prompting initiation of randomized trials.

Phase III trials were performed using an implanted pump (Infusaid 400) for intraarterial administration of FUDR at a dose of 0.2–0.3 mg/kg per day for 2 weeks every 4 weeks. In six randomized trials using this technique IAHC was compared with a control arm without IAHC (Chang et al.. 1987; Kemeny et al.. 1987; Hohn et al.. 1989; Martin et al.. 1990; Rougier et al.. 1992; Allen-Mersh et al.. 1994). In three of these trials, intravenous FUDR was administered via the same type of implanted pump in the control group (Chang et al.. 1987; Kemeny et al.. 1987; Hohn et al.. 1989). In another trial a monthly schedule of intravenous bolus 5FU was administered on 5 consecutive days to the control group (Martin et al.. 1990). In the last two trials IAHC was tested against ad libitum treatment (symptomatically intravenous 5FU) (Rougier et al.. 1992; Allen-Mersh et al.. 1994).

Results in terms of response rate clearly demonstrated the efficacy of IAHC but were less regarding survival (Table 1). In the four trials comparing intraarterial to intravenous FUDR or intravenous 5-FU, there was a two- to threefold increase in the *response rate*, a highly significant finding in all trials (Table 1). This result has been fully confirmed in the meta-analysis done by the Meta-analysis Group in Cancer (1996), which reported a response rate of 41% – complete remission (CR) 3% and partial remission (PR) 38% for the patients undergoing intraarterial treatment versus 14% (CR 2%, PR 12%) for the patients receiving intravenous chemotherapy ($p < 0.0001$).

Overall survival was also increased, but the results were more difficult to interpret. In four trials comparing intraarterial to intravenous chemotherapy this increase was not significant. Two of these trials incorporated a small number of patients and there was a clear lack of power (Chang et al.. 1987; Martin et al.. 1990). In the other two trials (Kemeny et al.. 1987; Hohn et al.. 1989) the patients allocated to the intravenous group were allowed to cross over and receive IAHC in case of tumor progression in the liver, which occurred in 31% and 60% of the cases, respectively, preventing survival comparisons between the IAHC and control groups. In contrast, the two Europe-

Table 1. Results of randomized trials comparing intraarterial hepatic chemotherapy (IAHC) with other nonintraarterial treatments

Study	No. of patients (total/eligible)	Protocol (IAHC vs. IV)	Response rate (%) (IAHC vs. IV)	Survival (months) (IAHC vs. IV)
Kemeny et al. (1987)	163/99	FUDR vs. FUDR	53 vs. 21*	17 vs. 12[a] (NS)
Chang et al. (1987)	64/50	FUDR vs. FUDR	62 vs. 17*	NS
Hohn et al. (1988)	143/117	FUDR vs. FUDR	42 vs. 10*	17 vs. 16[a] (NS)
Martin et al. (1990)	69/69	FUDR vs. 5FU	48 vs. 21*	12.6 vs. 10 (NS)
Rougier et al. (1992)	166/163	FUDR vs. 5FU ad libitum	49 vs. 13*	15 vs. 11**
Allen-Mersh et al. (1994)	100/100	FUDR vs. ad libitum symptomatic	–	13.0 vs. 7.5***
Meta-analysis Group in Cancer (1996)	654	FUDR/FUDR or 5FU or 0	41 vs. 14 $P<10^{-10}$	IAHC > control $P=0.0009$

5Fu, 5-fluorouracil, *FudR*, 5-fluor-2′deoxyuridine, *IV*, Intravenous; *NS*, not significant
[a] Crossover
*$p<0.05$; ** $p=0.02$; *** $p=0.03$

Table 2. Prognostic factor analysis for patients treated by IAHC: results of a multivariate analysis on 148 patients treated at the Institute Gustave Roussy (1984–1992)

Variable	Median survival[a] (months)	*P* (Cox model)
Clinical hepatomegaly: <5 vs. >5 cm	24 vs. 12	<0.00001
Replacement: <50% of healthy liver vs. >50%	21 vs. 11	<0.00001
CEA <100 vs. >100 ng/ml	25 vs. 12	<0.0001
Alkaline phosphatase <200 vs. >200 U/ml	23 vs. 14	<0.0001
Adequate arterial perfusion assessed by angioscintigraphy: yes vs. no	25 vs. 15	0.006

CEA, carcinoembryonic antigen

[a] Twenty percent of patients with good prognostic factors are alive at 3 years. Treatment protocols (5FU; FUDR; THP adriamycin+MMC) did not influence survival

an trials (Rougier et al.. 1992; Allen-Mersh et al.. 1994) specifically addressed the survival issue and compared IAHC with symptomatic treatment or intravenous bolus 5FU (the standard chemotherapy 10 years ago). These two studies involved a larger number of patients (166 and 100 respectively) and demonstrated that IAHC significantly improves overall survival ($p=0.02$ and $p=0.03$, respectively) and survival without progression (Table 1).

These studies have clearly established that IAHC effectively prolongs overall survival compared with symptomatic treatment or bolus 5FU. Indeed the relative value of IAHC compared with the more recent and efficient systemic chemotherapies (5FU plus leucovorin or methotrexate (or all three) or high-dose 5FU in weekly or biweekly 24- to 48-h infusions) is still unknown.

Many prognostic factors influenced survival in these trials, and we have performed a prognostic factor analysis using the Cox model (multivariate analysis) (Table 2). The survival rate is significantly influenced by three factors: the degree of hepatic involvement by the tumor (lower rate if it was more than 50%), the presence of clinical hepatomegaly (poorer if the lesion was more than 5 cm below the costal edge), and the quality of perfusion of the metastases (poorer if perfusion was poor) (Rougier et al.. 1991). Technical expertise importantly influenced the results as well. In the French trial survival was significantly better for patients treated in centers that had included more than 10 patients in their study group (Rougier et al.. 1992).

These results demonstrate that IAHC is an effective treatment especially for well selected patients. However, it is associated with some adverse events and has limits that must be discussed.

Adverse Events and Limits of IAHC

Toxicity. Toxicity, mainly hepatic, digestive, and systemic, has long been a limiting factor for IAHC. Hepatic and biliary toxicity depends on the type of drug and its administration schedule. It occurs with FUDR administered by continuous infusion over a 14-day period every 28 days via implanted pumps, and it is cumulative. Its frequency increases with the duration of the IAHC. For instance, in a French randomized trial, chemical hepatitis was reported in 35% of cases at 1 year and sclerosing cholangitis in about 25% (Rougier et al.. 1992). This toxicity is probably due to a direct toxic effect of the FUDR infusion in the terminal biliary arteries, resulting in chemical arteriolitis. Such toxicity can now be reduced: Careful biological follow-up, with IAHC interruption in case of an AP increase, or addition of dexamethasone (Rougier et al.. 1991; Kemeny et al.. 1994) and shortening the intraarterial perfusion from 14 days to 7 days every 28 days (Patt 1993 a) resulted in a significant decrease in the rate of sclerosing cholangitis. In contrast, IAHC with short 5FU infusions is associated with a low rate of hepatic toxicity or none (Rougier et al.. 1991); and other drugs [e.g., mitomycin C and TEP-rubicin (Rhone Poulenc Rorer Lab., Montrouge, France)], used in short infsions have no reported associated hepatic toxicity (Munck et al.. 1993).

Gastrointestinal toxicity was reported in 20–40% of eases, mainly gastroduodenal inflammation or ulceration, which occasionally leads to duodenal perforation. This toxicity is mainly due to extrahepatic perfusion, especially through nonligated pyloric arteries, and can be partly prevented by carefully dissecting the first part of the common hepatic artery at the time of catheter placement (Hohn et al.. 1986). *Arterial or catheter thrombosis* occurs during IAHC when subcutaneous access and discontinuous arterial perfusions are used. The risk is clearly related to the team's experience. In our practice the median life-span of a functional catheter has increased from 6.5 months 5 years ago (Meta-Analysis Group in Cancer 1996) to 12 months during our last study (Rougier et al.. 1996).

Extrahepatic Progression. Extrahepatic progression has about 50% of patients in the phase II and III trials when hepatic metastases are controlled by IAHC. Many authors have noted an unusual location of these extrahepatic metastases; for example cerebral and adrenal metastases have been reported in addition to lung and peritoneal metastases. This finding strongly supports combining intraarterial and intravenous chemotherapy. At present only one randomized trial has compared IAHC alone with IAHC plus intravenous 5FU; it demonstrated an advantage for the combination therapy in terms of survival without progression (Safi et al.. 1995). Additional trials using a more active systemic regimen are clearly needed.

Technical Expertise. When possible, surgical placement of the catheter seems preferable to placement under radiological control because it allows careful dissection of the gastroduodenal artery and common hepatic artery, cholecystectomy, ligation of the distal gastroduodenal artery, direct verification of the perfusion quality, and if necessary ligation of abnormal hepatic arteries (Elias et al.. 1987). From our experience it seems that the quality of perfusion, the rate of digestive complications, and probably the incidence of catheter thrombosis are dependent on the quality of surgical catheterization. In a French randomized trial the individual experience of the participating centers categorized into those with more than 10 randomized patients and those with fewer influenced significantly (independent of other prognostic factors) the overall survival rate (Rougier et al.. 1992). It is also interesting to note that in the U.K. study, in which 90% of the catheters were placed by the same surgeon, no catheterization failures were reported (Allen-Mersh et al.. 1994) compared with 11% in our study, in which 17 centers were involved (Rougier et al.. 1992). This finding is consistent with the results for 70 patients reported by Campbell et al.. (1993), who noted 37% technical complications for inexperienced surgeons versus 7% for experienced ones. For patients with normal anatomy the difference was even greater: 42% technical complications for inexperienced surgeons and none for experienced ones.

Cost. The cost of IAHC is high because of the equipment (especially the implantable pumps) and the expense associated with the surgical implantation of the pump and catheter. The cost of hospitalization must also be taken into account. If we compare patients treated with the implanted pump with those undergoing systemic chemotherapy administered weekly or five times a month in the outpatient clinic, the cost is equivalent after 6 months of treatment (without complications) because the patients with implanted pumps require only two outpatient visits per month (Patt 1993a). Thus IAHC performed by an experienced team in patients with favorable prognostic factors appears to be an acceptable therapeutic option.

Is There a Future for IAHC?

Development of New Drugs and New Protocols

Most studies have used fluoropyrimidines, which have favorable pharmacokinetic properties. Other agents, such as mitomycin C (MMC) and cis-platinum also have a favorable pharmacokinetic profile, and some studies have reported almost 30% response rates using monthly intraarterial injection of MMC after failure of IAHC using FUDR.

We have reported pharmacokinetic and experimental interest in an anthracycline, THP-adriamycin (TEP-Rubicin; Rhone Poulenc Rorer, Montrouge, France). Intraarterial hepatic administration of this agent in a rabbit model bearing VX2 tumors in the liver resulted in a 20-fold increase in intratumoral concentration of the drug compared to when it was administered intravenously and a 10-fold increase in tumor concentration compared to that in healthy liver. Based on these preclinical studies and a phase I study, the recommended dose for intraarterial administration was 75 mg/m^2 in a 30-min intraaterial hepatic infusion every 3 weeks (Munck et al.. 1993). A phase II trial was subsequently conducted in patients with liver metastases from colorectal cancer (LMCRC), and a 30% response rate was observed - an outstanding result if one considers the well established resistance of colorectal cancer (CRC) to anthrayclines.

Another development of IAHC is polychemotherapy. Kemeny et al.. (1993 a) reported interesting results using an FUDR + leucovorin combination, with a high response rate but high toxicity at the beginning of the study. In a randomized trial in pretreated patients these authors reported superiority of IAHC using the FUDR + MMC + BCNU combination over FUDR alone in terms of response rate (47% vs. 25%) and survival (median 19 months vs. 14 months). Thus polychemotherapy is an interesting way to improve IAHC efficacy, particularly as new active drugs have become available for colorectal cancer.

IAHC plus Effective Systemic Chemotherapy

The use of IAHC with fluoropyrimidines is associated with a low rate of systemic toxicity, a clear advantage. This findings illustrates the high hepatic clearance of drugs administered by the intraarterial route. It also illustrates the low systemic concentration of these drugs and the impossibility of obtaining a systemic effect. Since the recent demonstration of the efficacy of systemic chemotherapy in patients suffering from CRC metastases, the combined approach has seemed logical, but it has been only partly explored. Safi et al.. (1995) reported a significant increase in survival without disease progression when intraarterial and intravenous were combined, in contrast to intraarterial FUDR alone. We have reported encouraging results (Mahjoubi et al.. 1994) observed during a phase II study using the combination of intraarterial THP-adriamycin and intravenous 5FU + leucovorin. We also studied the efficacy of and tolerance to the combination of intraarterial MMC and systemic 5FU + leucovorin (Villanova et al.. 1996) and of intraarterial continuous infusion of high-dose 5FU for 4 days combined with systemic 5FU + leucovorin (Rougier et al.. 1996). Kemeny et al.. (1993 b) also reported encouraging results after combining intraarterial FUDR and systemic 5FU + leucovorin. These combinations of intraarterial hepatic and intravenous chemotherapy are well tolerated and effective in our experience (Rougier et al.. 1996; Villanova et al.. 1996), but it is too early to predict their impact on survival and extrahepatic progression, which must be further investigated in randomized trials.

Intraarterial hepatic chemotherapy is an active, useful technique in highly cases of LMCRC. The best indication is the presence of inoperable isolated liver metastases involving less than 50% of the liver (5–10% of cases). Using this indication and with optimal treatment techniques, there is hope of 50% 2-year survival and 5–14% 5-year survival. In some cases IAHC efficacy permits secondary resection, which was impossible prior to the introduction of this approach (Elias et al.. 1995). However, such secondary surgery is made difficult by changes in the healthy liver caused by the IAHC, which must be as short and as light as possible when such secondary surgery is planned.

Advantages of Isolated Liver Perfusion

Isolated liver perfusion (ILP) is a promising approach, combining intraarterial chemotherapy with extracorporeal extraction (Aigner et al.. 1988). It has been validated in an experimental model (Marinelli et al.. 1990). Experiences reported in this area clearly demonstrate that ILP is feasible using adequate anesthesia and an optimal technique.

The technique allows extracorporeal filtration, even after percutaneous placement of multichannel catheters, resulting in 80% extraction of circulating doxorubicin, 5FU or MMC, thereby allowing the use of high-dose chemotherapy. For other drugs, such as cis-diamminedichloroplatinum much less extraction (40%) is obtained.

In addition to this advantage in dose/intensity it is also possible to use biotherapy such as tumor necrosis factor, which cannot be applied by the systemic route because of its high toxicity. ILP can also be combined with hyperthermia, which improves the antitumor efficacy of some drugs.

The main limits of this technique are its complexity, potential toxicity (depending on the technique and the drugs used), and cost. Simplification with the use of posthepatic venous blood flow detoxification, without isolating the hepatic blood flow, has been developed; and objective antitumoral effects have been reported (Guadagni et al.. 1995).

Isolated liver perfusion has been reported useful for treating LMCRC (Aigner et al.. 1988), hepatocellular carcinoma, and liver metastases from ocular melanomas. The clinical value of ILP has not yet been demonstrated in comparative trials versus IAHC or systemic chemotherapy (or both) or other local treatment techniques, such as chemoembolization.

Therefore, the medical oncologist should restrict its use to randomized trials for unresectable LMCRC, with liver involvement of < 50% and it should be combined with systemic chemotherapy alone. Other indications (e.g., hepatocellular carcinoma, melanoma liver metastases, cholangiocarcinoma, and sarcoma liver metastases) are interesting fields of investigation but show no clear indications for ILP. Hence only prospective, multicenter trials, if possible with randomization against "standard treatment," can be recommended.

Conclusions

Locoregional treatments of unresectable liver tumors are efficient and have not been replaced by the development of active systemic treatment. Their development in combination with systemic treatment methods, when they are efficient, is logical and would potentially benefit the patients, allowing better local and systemic control of the tumor.

The efficacy of IAHC is now established for LMCRC, which is not the case for ILP. ILP is presently between the experimental and the standard stage of development and requires multiple prospective trials before it can be accepted by medical oncologists. Owing to the technical complexity and the cost of this method, only common and multidisciplinary research protocols can help define precisely the best indications for ILP.

References

Aigner KR, Walther H, Link KH (1988) Isolated liver perfusion with MMC/5-FU: Surgical technique, pharmacokinetics, clinical results. Contrib Oncol 29:229–246

Allen-Mersh TG, Earlam S, Fordy C, Abrams K, Houghton J (1994) Quality of life and survival with continuous hepatic-artery floxiuridine infusion for colorectal liver metastases. Lancet 344:1255–1260

Breedis C, Young C (1954) The blood supply of neoplasm in the liver. Am J Pathol 30:969–974

Campbell KA, Burns RC, Sitzmann JV, Lipsett PA, Grochow LB, Niederhuber JE (1993) Regional chemotherapy devices: effect of experience and anatomy on complications. J Clin Oncol 11:822–826

Chang AE, Schneider PD, Sugarbaker PH, Simpson C, Culnane M, Steinberg SM (1987) A prospective randomized trial of regional versus systemic continuous 5-fluorodeoxyuridine chemotherapy in the treatment of colorectal liver metastases. Ann Surg 206:685–693

Chen GHG, Gross JF (1980) Intra-arterial infusion of anticancer drugs: theoretic aspects of drug delivery and review of responses. Cancer Treat Rep 64:31–40

Elias D, Lasser P, Rougier P (1987) A simplified surgical technical procedure for intra-arterial chemotherapy in secondary liver cancer: experience in 50 patients. Eur J Surg Oncol 13:441–448

Elias D, Lasser P, Rougier P, Ducreux M, Bognel C, Roche A (1995) Frequency, technical aspects, results and indications of major hepatectomy alter prolonged intra-arterial hepatic chemotherapy for initially unresectable hepatic tumors. J Am Coll Surg 180:213–219

Ensminger WD, Gyves JW (1983) Regional chemotherapy of neoplastic diseases. Pharmacol Ther 21:277–293

Hohn DC, Rayner AA, Economou JS, Ignoffo RJ, Lewis BJ, Stagg RJ (1986) Toxicities and complications of implanted pump hepatic arterial and intravenous floxuridine infusion. Cancer 57:465–470

Hohn DC, Stagg RJ, Friedman MA, Hannigan JF, Rayner A, Ignoffo RJ et al. (1989) A randomized trial of continuous intravenous versus hepatic intraarterial floxiuridine in patients with colorectal cancer metastatic to the liver: the Northern California Oncology Group trial. J Clin Oncol 7:1646–1654

Kemeny N (1992) Is hepatic infusion of chemotherapy effective treatment for liver metastases? Yes. In: DeVita VT, Hellman S, Rosenberg SA (eds) Important advances in oncology. Lippincott, Philadelphia pp 207–228

Kemeny N, Daly J, Reichman B, Geller N, Botet J, Oderman P (1987) Intrahepatic or systemic infusion of fluorodeoxyuridine in patients with liver metastases from colorectal carcinoma. Ann Intern Med 107:459–465

Kemeny N, Cohen A, Seiter K, Conti JA, Sigurdson ER, Tao Y et al. (1993a) Randomized trial of hepatic arterial floxuridine, mitomycin, and carmustine versus floxuridine alone in previously treated patients with liver metastases from colorectal cancer. J Clin Oncol 11:330–335

Kemeny N, Conti JA, Sigurdson E, Cohen A, Seiter K, Lincer R et al. (1993b) A pilot study of hepatic artery floxuridine combined with systemic 5-fluorouracil and leucovorin. Cancer 71:1964–1971

Kemeny N, Conti JA, Cohen A, Campana P, Huang Y, Shi WJ et al. (1994) Phase II study of hepatic arterial floxuridine, leucovorin, and dexamethasone for unresectable liver metastases from colorectal carcinoma. J Clin Oncol 12:2288–2295

Mahjoubi R, Ychou M, Ducreux M, Seitz JF, Colin P, Olivier et al. (1994) Multicentric phase II trial of intrahepatic arterial (HAI) pirarubiem (P) and systemic 5 fluorouracil (5FU) + leucovorin (LV) for liver metastases (LM) from colorectal cancer (CRC). Proc Am Soc Clin Oncol 13:223

Marinelli A, Pons DHA, Vreeken JAC, Nagesser SK, Maurits de Brauw L, Franken H, Tjaden UR, van de Velde CJH (1990) Pharmacological evaluation of isolated liver perfusion with high-dose 5-fluorouracil and mitomycin C in pigs. Reg Cancer Treat 3:192–196

Martin JK, O'Connell MJ, Wieand HS, Fitzgibbons RJ, Mailliard JA, Rubin J et al. (1990) Intra-arterial floxuridine vs systemic fluorouracil for hepatic metastases from colorectal cancer: A randomized trial. Arch Surg 125:1022–1027

Meta-analysis Group in Cancer (1996) Reappraisal of arterial infusion in the treatment of nonresectable liver metastases from colorectal cancer. J Natl Cancer Inst 88:252–258

Munck JN, Riggi M, Rougier P, Chabot GG, Ramirez LH, Zhao Z et al. (1993) Pharmacokinetic and pharmacodynamic advantages of pirarubicin over adriamycin alter intraarterial hepatic administration in the rabbit VX2 tumor model. Cancer Res 53:1550–1554

O'Connell MJ (1992) Is hepatic infusion of chemotherapy effective treatment for liver metastases? No. In: DeVita VT, Hellman S, Rosenberg SA (eds) Important advances in oncology. Lippincott, Philadelphia, pp 229–234

Patt Y (1993a) Regional hepatic arterial chemotherapy for colorectal cancer metastatic to the liver: the controversy continues. J Clin Oncol 11:815–819

Patt Y (1993b) Hepatic artery chemotherapy for colorectal liver metastases: yet more controversy. J Clin Oncol 11:2053–2054

Rougier P, Ducreux M, Pignon JP, Elias D, Tigaud JM, Lumbroso J et al. (1991) Prognostic factors in patients with liver metastases from colorectal carcinoma treated with discontinuous intra-arterial hepatic chemotherapy. Eur J Cancer 10:1226–1230

Rougier P, Laplanche A, Huguier M, Hay JM, Ollivier JM, Escat J et al. (1992) Hepatic arterial infusion of floxuridine in patients with liver metastases from colorectal carcinoma: long-term results of a prospective randomized trial. J Clin Oncol 10:1112–1118

Rougier P, Milan C, Lazorthes F, Fourtanier G, Partensky C, Gouzi JL et al. (1995) Unresected hepatic metastases from colorectal cancer: prognostic factor analysis from a prospective study on 544 cases from the Fondation Francaise de Cancerologie Digestive (FFCD). Br J Surg 82:1397–1400

Rougier P, Ducreux M, Ychou M, Duffour J, Ramos G, Elias D et al. (1996) Intra-arterial chemotherapy (IAHC) using mitomycin C (MMC) combined to intra-venous chemotherapy (IVC) using 5FU + folinic acid (FA) for hepatic metastases from colorectal cancer (HMCRC). Proc Am Soc Clin Oncol 15:206

Safi F, Hepp G, Link KH, Beger HG (1995) Simultaneous adjuvant regional and systemic chemotherapy after resection of liver metastases of colorectal cancer. Proc Am Soc Clin Oncol 14:217

Villanova G, Ducreux M, Samelis G, Lumbroso J, Lasser P, Elias D, Rougier P (1996) Chimiothérapie intraartérielle hépatique (CIAH) par 5-fluorouracile (5-FU) en perfusion continue (PC) associé à un traitement intraveineux (IV) par 5-FU et acide folinique. Bull Cancer (Paris) 83:439

Indication for Isolated Hyperthermic Liver Perfusion: A Surgeon's View

T. Scherstén

University of Göteborg, Sahlgrenska Hospital, Department of Surgery,
S-41345 Göteborg, Sweden

We cannot continue doing things
merely because we know how to do
Sir Theodor Fox

Abstract

Isolated hyperthermic liver perfusion is a transitional therapy, i.e. a therapy between evidence based, standard therapy and experimental therapy. It appears to provide distinct benefits in a number of situations but the scientific evidence is still incomplete. In our view the present indications for use of isolated hyperthermic perfusion of the liver are:

- to gain more knowledge;
- nonresectable liver metastases without proven extrahepatic growth from: uveal melanoma, colorectal carcinoma, and ovarian cancer;
- symptoms related to hepatic metastases from endocrine tumors. A multicenter study aimed at gaining more knowledge is recommended.

Introduction

Indications for use of a technique address such issues as for whom for what, and how much of a given therapy should be used – issues covered by most scientific clinical studies in the medical literature. Although almost all medical therapies have a range of possible applications for treating various symptoms and diseases, it is not always possible to define this range clearly or to set boundaries for their use. One reason is that we have different categories of therapies with quite different objectives. Consequently, we must determine the category into which a certain therapy falls before we can discuss its indications.

Categories of Therapy

In my view, there are four therapeutic categories: evidence-based therapy, emotion-based therapy, experimental therapy, and transitional therapy.

Evidence-Based Therapy

The criteria for evidence-based, standard therapies are (1) established indications of use; (2) specified outcomes of care, where risks and benefits are well defined; (3) standardized requirements of application (skills staff, facilities for proper use); and (4) articulated criteria for learning and certification.

Established indications of use should be based on randomized controlled trials and on the best meta-analyses (of the kind performed by the Cochrane Collaborating Centers). The only exception is when a new therapy diseases, such as heart or liver transplantation in patients with end-stage heart or liver diseases.

When *outcomes* are enumerated it must be possible to denote a particular therapy as standard. In the past the outcomes analyzed were restricted to specific biological changes, whereas in more recent times outcomes have been assessed, in addition, with respect to the functional and subjective effects of a therapy as the patient experiences them (i.e., quality of life). The physician and patient should have a clear understanding of what risks must be taken for the benefit gained. This knowledge eases the burden of action and enhances the efficiency of standard therapy.

Standardized requirements of application focus on the manner in which a given therapy is applied. It *involves a clear* definition of the skill of the medical staff who apply the therapy and the necessary facilities, including other medical specialties, for safe and proper use of the technology.

Criteria for learning and certification must be clearly defined. When setting these criteria, answers to the following question may be helpful: How many hours of training are needed, or how many patients must be seen, to apply the technology? Who should teach this field? What are appropriate educational venues? Who should oversee the certification process?

Emotional Based Therapy

Emotion-based therapy is unfortunately rather commonly applied. This type of therapy has no scientifically established indications and is not used under a research protocol. It is more a prescription based on the doctor's embarrassment when he or she has nothing to offer. There may be no effective therapy available, and it is too difficult for the doctor to inform the patient about the situation. This method avoids dealing with the patients problem for the moment and must be considered unworthy of modern medicine.

Experimental Therapy

Experimental therapy is characterized by uncertainty. The only indication for its use is the collection of information to gain knowledge. Experimental therapy can therefore be applied only within the context of a specified research protocol formulated to answer questions about its efficacy and safety or about its economic, social, and ethical implications. The protocol is known as technology assessment and is an established discipline with the aim of developing a synthesis of information by integrating biological, clinical, economic, and social factors. Methods and the relevant literature can be marshaled to produce the wider range of knowledge needed to establish the experimental therapy as standard.

Transitional Therapy

Transitional therapy lies somewhere between standard and experimental treatments. Any therapy of this type evolves when an experimental therapy appears to provide distinct benefits, but studies on it are incomplete. Transitional therapy is also generated when a therapy that has been approved as standard for given applications is used to treat problems for which it was not tested initially. Another situation arises when new side effects are discovered after long-term use of a standard therapy.

If a transitional therapy is the only hope for patients in desperate need of help, there is significant pressure to apply it as a nonexperimental therapy. Physicians and scientific bodies confront a difficult question when facing this issue. If a doctor decides to act when knowledge is inadequate, he or she risks doing more harm than good. Hence it must be decided whether the risk of harm to the patient outweighs the risk of treating the illness with conventional methods. The fact that patients ask for and consent to the treatment does not relieve the doctor of ethical or legal responsibility – it simply gives permission to initiate action.

Conclusions

Isolated hyperthermic liver perfusion must be considered a transitional therapy. It appears to provide distinct benefits in a number of situations. At present it seems prudent to use the technique for the following indications: (1) to gain knowledge; (2) to treat nonresectable metastases without proved extrahepatic growth from uveal melanoma, colorectal cancer, or ovarian cancer; and (3) to alleviate symptoms related to hepatic metastases from endocrine tumors. Because there are comparatively few such cases seen at single centers, I recommend that we develop a common research protocol to be used in a multicenter study. Although the technique is a "thing of beauty," it would be well to remember that:

The reason why men prefer beauty over brains
is that they can see better than they can think.
Fawcett

II. Technique/Anaesthesia

Asanguineous Isolated Hyperthermic Perfusion of the Liver: Results of an Experimental Study in Pigs

H. Lang[1], S. Nadalin[1], L. Moreno[2], A. Thyen[1], S. R. Shehata[1], P. Flemming[2], K. J. Oldhafer[1], and R. Pichlmayr † [1]

[1] Klinik für Abdominal- und Transplantationschirurgie, Medizinische Hochschule Hannover, Carl-Neuberg-Strasse 1, D-30625 Hannover, Germany
[2] Institut für Pathologie, Medizinische Hochschule Hannover, Carl-Neuberg-Strasse 1, D-30625 Hannover, Germany

Abstract

Asanguineous hyperthermic liver perfusion was performed in five and seven pigs for 30 and 45 min respectively. Laboratory data, including changes of liver enzyme levels and results of liver function tests, as well as morphological alterations of liver structure, were compared with data from a 45-min oxygenated hyperthermic liver perfusion. In the groups undergoing asanguineous liver perfusion survival was four of five and five of seven animals. In the oxygenated group six of seven pigs survived. Liver enzymes and function tests in the two groups with a 45-min perfusion time were not significantly different. All enzyme and laboratory test values returned to normal within 1 week. Similarly morphological changes were reversible within 1 week. The results suggest that asanguineous isolated hyperthermic liver perfusion up to 45 min is feasible without damage to liver tissue.

Introduction

Isolated organ perfusion with chemotherapy is a well-established practice in the treatment of irresectable soft tissue sarcomas and melanomas of the extremities (Eggermont et al. 1996). The concept of isolated organ perfusion was to allow the application of high doses of chemotherapy, simultaneously avoiding or at least reducing the systemic side effects of the drugs. Isolated hyperthermic liver perfusion (IHLP) was introduced as a locoregional therapy for disseminated liver cancer more than 30 years ago (Ausman 1961). It has been shown that temperatures above 42 °C (high-dose hyperthermia 42.1–44.0 °C) can irreversibly damage malignant cells. However, at this temperature, severe side effects have been reported in normal hepatic parenchyma. At lower temperatures, hyperthermia is less effective but, in combination with cytotoxic agents, a synergistic antineoplastic effect can be achieved without the risks of hyperthermia-induced liver damage (Skibba and Collins 1978).

So far, both isolated liver perfusion and isolated limb perfusion have been performed with oxygenated perfusates (Eggermont et al. 1996; Hafström et al. 1994). However, depending on the chemotherapeutic drugs administered in the perfusion circuit, hypoxia or anoxia might enhance the antineoplastic efficacy of this treatment (Senzer 1989). In isolated liver perfusion the use of an hypoxic or even anoxic perfusate is limited by the risk of ischemic damage to normal hepatic tissue and especially to hepatic sinusoids. From liver surgery it is known that hepatic vascular occlusion can be tolerated for more than 1 h under normothermic or mild hypothermic conditions (Hannoun et al. 1993). However, up till now only few data exist regarding the tolerance of normal hepatic parenchyma to anoxic and hyperthermic perfusion.

The purpose of the presented study is to evaluate the tolerance of normal liver tissue to anoxic perfusion with additional application of mild hyperthermia. One aim was also to compare functional and structural changes of hepatic tissue after oxygenated perfusion with alterations of liver function caused by anoxic perfusion.

Material and Methods

The experiments were performed in a standardized animal model (Lang et al. 1997). Nineteen pigs (German landrace) with a body weight of between 25 and 40 kg were divided into three groups: A ($n=7$) B ($n=5$) and C ($n=7$). In group A (control group) oxygenated IHLP was performed for 45 min. In groups B and C isolated anoxic perfusions were performed for 30 and 45 min, respectively. The protocol for the experiments was approved by the regional research committee for the care and use of laboratory animals.

Operative Procedure

Total vascular isolation of the liver was achieved after complete mobilization of the liver and dissection of the hepatoduodenal ligament, with ligation of all arterial branches to the stomach and small intestine (with the exception of the gastroduodenal artery). Special attention was paid to tying all diaphragmatic veins to avoid systemic leakage of perfusate. A cavo-porto-jugular veno-venous bypass was inserted to maintain hemodynamic stability during isolated perfusion. The portal vein, the gastroduodenal artery and the infrahepatic inferior vena cava were cannulated with special catheters. Liver perfusion was performed via the hepatic artery and the portal vein, with the caval vein serving as venous outflow tract. Total vascular isolation was completed by clamping the suprahepatic inferior vena cava and the common hepatic artery proximal to the gastroduodenal artery. To avoid leakage of perfusate into the systemic circulation the bile duct was temporarily obstructed with a tourniquet to close all accompanying vessels.

Perfusion Circuit

The perfusion circuit consisted of a recirculating perfusion system with an integrated heat exchanger (Bio-Cal 370 Bio-Medicus, Medtronic, Bad Homburg, Germany) and two roller pumps, as well as a biopump. A minipulsator in the portal line guaranteed a continuous and non-pulsating portal inflow. For oxygenation in group A a membrane-oxygenator (Minimax CB 1381 Hollow Fiber Oxygenator, Bio-Medicus, Medtronic, Bad Homburg, Germany) was integrated additionally (Fig. 1).

In groups B and C (anoxic perfusion groups) the perfusate consisted of 1000 ml Ringer's solution and 750 ml oxypolygelatine (Gelifundol), as well als 5000 IU of heparin. In these two groups a prewash-out (500 ml NaCl 0.9%) of the liver via the portal vein was performed in order to rinse the trapped blood out of the liver. In group A (control group, oxygenated perfusion) the perfusate consisted of the same amount of Ringer's solution (1000 ml) but only 500 ml oxypolygelatine. In addition 250 ml of the pig's own blood (plus the trapped intrahepatic blood), as well as 5000 IU of heparin were added to the perfusate.

Total perfusion time was 45 min in groups A and C and 30 min in group B. The perfusion was carried out at a mean inflow temperature of 41.2 °C (range 40.5–42.0 °C). The mean arterial and portal perfusion pressures were adjusted to between 40 and 60 mmHg and 20 and 25 mmHg, respectively. The mean inflow rates were 130 ml/min for the artery and 500 ml/min for the portal vein. Table 1 summarizes the perfusion parameters.

Before reperfusion, the liver was washed out with Ringer's solution (2000 ml) and 500 ml dextran in all groups. Then the clamps on the hepatic artery and the suprahepatic vena cava were removed and arterial reperfusion started. Next portal blood flow was restored through an end-to-end anastomosis and, finally, the infrahepatic vena cava was reconstructed in the same way.

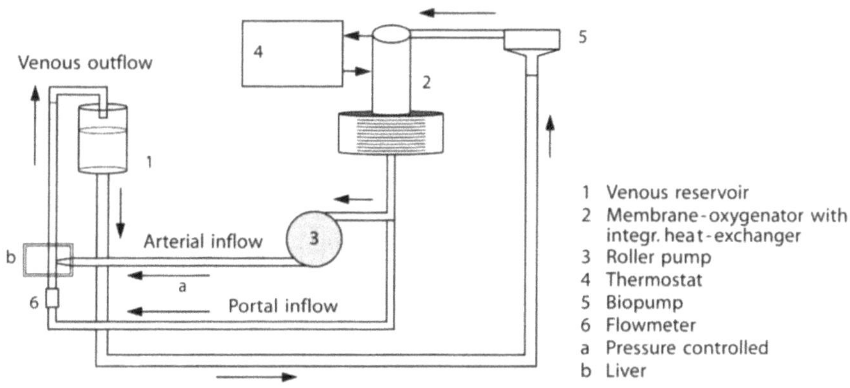

Fig. 1. Scheme of perfusion circuit

Table 1. Perfusion parameters

Perfusate temperature	
Inflow	41.2 °C (40.5–42.0 °C)
Outflow	39.5 °C (38.3–40.8 °C)
Mean portal perfusion	
Pressure 20–25 mmHg	
Flow 500 ml/min	
Mean arterial perfusion	
Pressure 40–60 mmHg	
Flow 130 ml/min	

Monitoring

Vital parameters (heart rate, central venous pressure, blood pressure, blood gas analysis, serum concentration of sodium and potassium) were monitored continuously during the operation. Ringer's solution and plasma expanders were used for fluid substitution. Electrolytes and acid-base disorders were corrected with calcium gluconate, potassium chloride and sodium bicarbonate. During perfusion, the liver temperature was monitored continuously with two needle probes in the right and left liver lobes.

End-points of the Study

Blood samples were drawn before operation, 4 h after reperfusion and on postoperative days 1, 3, 5 and 7. Liver biopsies for histologic and electronic microscopic evaluation were taken before perfusion, 1 h after reperfusion and at the end of the observation period (1 week) or immediately after death if a pig died during the observation period.

The three groups were compared with regard to mortality and morbidity, alterations of liver enzyme levels and function test results, as well as changes in liver morphology.

Results

In all pigs a stable liver perfusion with a mean liver temperature of 40.5 °C (left lobe 40.3 °C, right lobe 40.8 °C) could be achieved after 15 min. Perfusate pH ranged between 6.8 and 7.1 in the anoxic groups and 7.2 and 7.5 in the oxygenated group.

Survival rates were 6/7 in group A, 4/5 in group B and 5/7 in group C. In group A the cause of death was a portal vein thrombosis, which occurred after re-anastomosis after an initial stenosis of the reconstructed portal vein. In group B one pig died due to severe systemic hypotension and cardiopulmonary failure. In group C, one death was caused by cardiopulmonary failure within 12 h after reperfusion. In this group, a second pig died on the first postoperative day. It had an uneventful initial postoperative course but its general condition deteriorated rapidly 24 h after operation. Pathology revealed a severe necrotizing pancreatitis as the most probable cause of death.

The total vascular occlusion times are summarized in Table 2. For groups B and C the duration of arterial clamping was identical to the period of total anoxia of the liver. Total vascular occlusion time minus arterial clamping time represents the time of reduced oxygen supply (hepatic artery perfused, portal vein clamped). In group A (oxygenated perfusion of the liver) the period of reduced oxygen supply is given by the total vascular occlusion times minus 45 min. This is the time which was required for insertion of the portal branch of the veno-venous bypass and for the anastomosis of the portal vein after liver perfusion. In groups A, B and C total clamping times of the hepatic artery were 51, 34 and 50 min, respectively. For the portal vein the total occlusion times (median value) were 81, 58 and 77 min, respectively. The longer occlusion time of the portal vein in comparison to the hepatic artery is explained by the insertion of a cavo-porto-jugular veno-venous bypass and the time required for reconstruction of the portal vein after the perfusion. For groups B and C arterial and portal vein clamping time was the same in surviving and non-surviving pigs. In group A the portal occlusion time in the only non-surviving pig was much longer because the portal vein anastomosis had to be done twice.

Laboratory data showed very similar results for groups A and C, the two groups perfused for 45 min. In all groups transaminase levels peaked on the 1st (AST) and 3rd (ALT) postoperative day, respectively (Figs. 2, 3). Enzyme levels did not exceed 700 U/l and normalized within the observation period. In all groups, serum lactate concentrations increased during the isolation period of the liver with a maximum at 30 min after reperfusion up to almost ten times the normal value. In all surviving pigs lactate levels returned to normal within 1 day (Fig. 4). Cholestasis parameters revealed only minimal changes. While there were almost no changes in serum bilirubin levels in any of the surviving

Table 2. Vascular occlusion

Vessel	Clamping time (min)		
	Oxygenated 45 min	Anoxic 30 min	Anoxic 45 min
Arterial			
Total	51	34	50
Surviving	51	33	48
Dead	51	35	51
Portal			
Total	81	58	77
Surviving	77	53	77
Dead	90	63	78

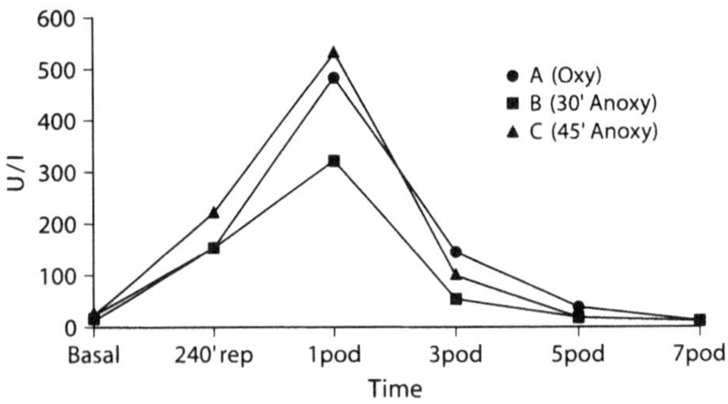

Fig. 2. Changes of transaminase levels (AST; pod, postoperative day; rep, reperfusion

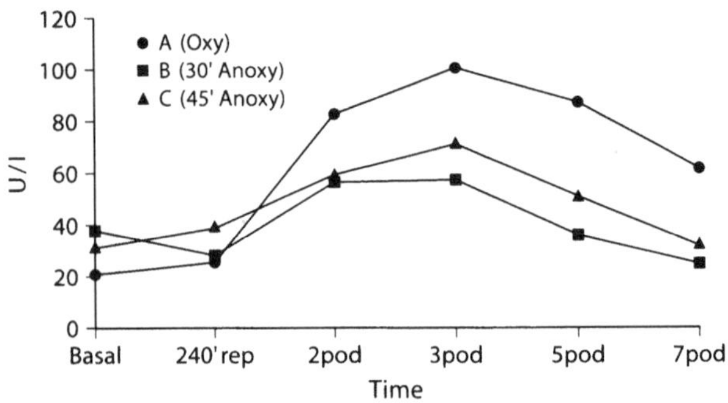

Fig. 3. Changes of transaminase levels (ALT)

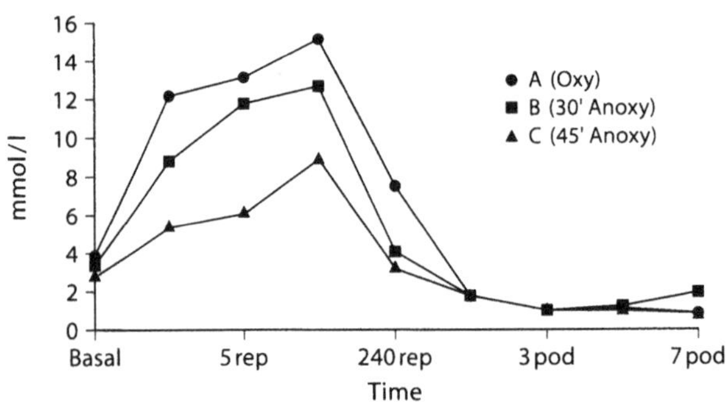

Fig. 4. Serum lactate levels

pigs, measurement of alkaline phosphatase showed a slight increase after perfusion. At the end of the observation period this enzyme also decreased to normal values. The Quick's test as a marker of the liver function showed a minimum level 4 h after reperfusion but completely normalized within 1 postoperative week. For all examined laboratory data there was no significant difference between surviving pigs of groups A and C.

Histology and electronic microscopy of the biopsy material taken 1 hour after reperfusion revealed vacuolization and edematous swelling of hepatocytes in all study groups. Similar to the laboratory tests histologic examination revealed no evidence of damage to the biliary tree.

Specimens taken at autopsy 1 week after perfusion demonstrated in almost all probes normal liver tissue with only a few areas of focal regeneration. Damage to the biliary tree could not be found in any of the biopsies taken 1 week after perfusion.

Discussion

The liver is supposed to be very sensitive to hypoxia and ischemic damage, especially under normothermic conditions such as during a Pringle's maneuver. However, the experimental data of Nordlinger and co-workers showed that prolonged hepatic ischemia for up to 2 h could be survived if splanchnic decompression was performed. In these animal experiments, a 3-h vascular occlusion of the hepatic hilus was lethal to all pigs (Nordlinger et al. 1980). These experimental data have been confirmed to some extent by recent reports on liver surgery with vascular occlusion exceeding 1 h (Hannoun et al. 1993; Huguet et al. 1978). It is noteworthy that, during vascular occlusion, liver temperature is lowered to hypothermic values. This decrease of liver temperature is thought to have a protective effect on liver tissue by reducing the hepatic oxygen requirement. Thus, these data on occlusion of the hepatic hilus obviously do not allow conclusions to be made about the tolerance of liver tissue to hyperthermia in combination with hypoxia or anoxia.

The potential therapeutic effect of hyperthermia on malignant tumor cells has been demonstrated both in vitro and in vivo. The temperatures required for irreversible damage to tumor cells range above 42 °C. However, it has been shown that temperatures higher than 42.0 °C also have adverse effects on normal tissue, especially on liver tissue. In animal experiments, as well as in rare clinical observations, the hepatotoxic side effects of high-dose hyperthermia (>42 °C) could be confirmed by several authors (Horikawa et al. 1994; Skibba and Collins 1978). At lower temperatures (mild or moderate hyperthermia) there is only a minor antineoplastic effect but, in combination with chemotherapy, a synergistic cytotoxic potential can be achieved. In addition, the antineoplastic efficacy of heat and chemotherapy might even be enhanced by ischemia, which alone already has a proven antitumoral effect (i.e., in case of hepatic artery ligation for neuroendocrine hepatic metastases). This has been suggested by preclinical and clinical studies (Hill and Denekamp 1978; Moertel et al. 1994).

The literature yields discordant reports about the ideal temperature at which to achieve a synergistic therapeutic effect, as well as avoiding damage to normal liver tissue (Horikawa et al. 1994; Sindelair 1984; Van de Velde et al. 1986). We used a mean inflow temperature of 41.2 °C and reached a mean intrahepatic temperature of 40.5 °C. At this temperature, Horikawa and co-workers suggest a synergistic effect of chemotherapy and hyperthermia (Horikawa et al. 1994). The fact that the right liver lobe showed different temperatures from the left lobe is consistent with findings of other investigators (Adam et al. 1987). This is mainly explained by the location of the right lobe under the right abdominal wall and the chest and the less favorable ratio of volume and surface of the left lobe, resulting in a higher temperature dispersion.

Hyperthermic hypoxic liver perfusion has been studied experimentally in rats and dogs. The results of these experiments suggest that there are enormous variations in the tolerance of liver tissue to hyperthermic anoxic perfusion (Adam et al. 1987; Horikawa et al. 1994). Since the hepatic physiology in pigs is similar to the human, we chose the pig model for isolated perfusions. To avoid vascular and parenchymal damage to the liver due to the perfusion it is very important to apply physiological conditions in terms of perfusion pressure and flow pattern. In our model this was achieved by use of roller pumps and a biopump. Thus, the influence of perfusion-related damage could be minimized.

Our model could show that asanguineous liver perfusion for up to 45 min is feasible without damage to liver tissue. In addition the results of the laboratory data and the histological findings indicate that normal liver parenchyma can even tolerate the combination of anoxia and mild hyperthermia. All damage to the liver was almost completely reversible within 1 week after perfusion. The results of asanguineous and oxygenated perfusion are difficult to compare because, in the oxygenated pigs, hemoglobin levels of the perfusate were not physiological by the fact that only 250 ml blood plus the trapped intrahepatic blood were added to 1500 ml of perfusate. Thus, the "anemic" condition of the perfusate in the oxygenated group may be responsible for the very similar data from this group and the asanguineous perfused group. Nevertheless, it could also be demonstrated that an asanguineous hyperthermic perfusion of the liver (mild hyperthermia) can be tolerated by normal hepatic parenchyma.

In a first clinical study, Horikawa and co-workers could show that a hyperthermic hypoxic liver perfusion at an inflow temperature of between 42 °C and 43 °C for 30 min via the portal vein can be tolerated by livers during hepatic resection or immediately after hepatic resection. In their series even the administration of chemotherapeutic drugs (either mitomycin C or cisplatin) did not lead to liver damage. Our experiments suggest that it should be possible to extend the asanguineous period to up to 45 min in order to increase the antineoplastic efficacy of the perfusion. However, in our experiments, we did not add chemotherapeutic agents to the perfusion circuit. Thus, before clinical use of an anoxic/hypoxic liver perfusion for 45 min for treatment of irresectable liver tumors, further studies will have to assess the tolerance of liver tissue to the combination of hyperthermia plus hypoxia with chemotherapy.

Acknowledgment. This study was supported by the Paul-Blümel-Stiftung, Hannover

References

Adam R, Poggi L, Capron M, Morin J, Gigou M, Miramand JC, Szekely AM, Houssin D (1987) Asanguineous isolated hyperthermic in vivo perfusion of the liver in the rat. Eur Surg Res 19:366–374

Ausman RK (1961) Development of a technique for isolated perfusion of the liver. N State J Med 61:3993–3997

Eggermont AMM, Schraffordt Koops H, Klausner JM, Kroon BBR, Schlag PM, Lienard D, v Geel AN, Hoekstra HJ, Meller I, Nieweg OE, Kettelhack C, Ben-Ari G, Pector JC, Lejeune FJ (1996) Isolated limb perfusion with Tumor Necrosis Factor and Melphalan for limb salvage in 186 patients with locally advanced soft tissue extremity sarcomas. Ann Surg 224:756–765

Hafström LR, Holmberg SB, Naredi PLJ, Lindner PG, Bengtsson A, Tidebrant G, Schersten TSO (1994) Isolated hyperthermic liver perfusion with chemotherapy for liver malignancy. Surg Oncol 3:103–108

Hannoun L, Borie D, Delva E, Jones D, Vaillant JC, Nordlinger B, Parc R (1993) Liver resection with normothermic ischaemia exceeding 1 h. Br J Surg 80:1161–1165

Hill SA, Denekamp J (1978) The effect of vascular occlusion on the thermal sensitization of a mouse tumor. Br J Radiol 51:997–1002

Horikawa M, Nakajima Y, Kido K, Ko S, Ohashi K, Nakano H (1994) Simple method of hyperthermo-chemo-hypoxic isolated liver perfusion for hepatic metastases. World J Surg 18:845–851

Huguet C, Nordlinger B, Galopin JJ, Bloch P, Gallot D (1978) Normothermic hepatic vascular exclusion for extensive hepatectomy. Surg Gynecol Obstet 147:689–693

Lang H, Nadalin S, Flemming P, Thyen A, Moreno L, Oldhafer K, Pichlmayr R (1997) Tierexperimentelle Untersuchungen zur isolierten Leberperfusion mit Tumornekrosefaktor alpha. Langenbecks Arch Chir Suppl Kongressbd 339–343

Moertel CG, Johnson M, McKusick MA, Martin JK, Nagorney DM, Kvols LK, Rubin J, Kunselman S (1994) The management of patients with advanced carcinoid tumors and islet cell carcinomas. Ann Intern Med 120:302–309

Nordlinger B, Douvin D, Javaudin L, Bloch P, Aranda A, Boschat M, Huguet C (1980) An experimental study after two hours of normothermic hepatic ischemia. Surg Gynecol Obstet 150:859–864

Senzer NN (1989) Hyperthermia: chemotherapeutic and biologic response modifications. Strahlenther Onkol 165:729–733

Sindelair WF (1984) Method of isolation-perfusion of the liver in pig. Am Surg 50:557–563

Skibba JL, Collins FG (1978) Effect of temperature on biochemical function in the isolated perfused rat liver. J Surg Res 24:435–441

Van de Velde CJH, Kothuis BJL, Barenbrug HWM, Jongejan N, Runia RD, De Braw LM, Zwaveling A (1986) A successful technique of in vivo isolated liver perfusion in pigs. J Surg Res 41:593–599

Hyperthermo-Chemo-Hypoxic Isolated Liver Perfusion for Hepatic Metastases: A Possible Adjuvant Approach

Y. Nakajima, M. Horikawa, T. Kin, T. Ohyama, H. Kanehiro, M. Hisanaga, K. Nishio, M. Nagao, M. Sho, T. Yamada, K. Ohashi, S. Ko, and H. Nakano

First Department of Surgery, Nara Medical University, 840 Shijo-cho, Kashihara, Nara 634, Japan

Abstract

As a possible intraoperative adjuvant approach to treating hepatic metastases we developed a method of hyperthermo-chemo-hypoxic isolated liver perfusion in combination with hepatic resection. This method was applied to 11 patients with colorectal hepatic metastases between 1992 and 1995. One patient died on postoperative day 14 of hepatic failure (9% mortality), the cause of which was a liver temperature that reached 42.9 °C, which seems to be the maximum limit for thermal toxic effect on the human liver. The other 10 patients tolerated the perfusion well, with mild hepatic and no systemic toxicity after minor or even major hepatic resection; the serum aminotransferase and total bilirubin levels returned to normal levels by postoperative day 14. Only one of eight patients (13%) for whom cytotoxic drugs were added to the perfusate (mitomycin C 10 μg/ml or cisplatin 2 μg/ml) had hepatic recurrence by 19 months after the perfusion (mean follow-up 25.8 months; median 23 months; range 8–57 months). Two patients were alive with no evidence of disease at 13 and 57 months, respectively after the perfusion; the other five patients had postperfusion extrahepatic recurrences (median: 19 months; range 7–20 months). In contrast, hepatic metastases recurred 7 and 20 months after the perfusion, respectively, in the two patients not given a cytotoxic drug.

Introduction

Although liver metastasis from colorectal cancer is now actively resected, recurrence of hepatic metastases following liver resection is a well-known clinical situation. Tumor recurrence has been demonstrated in 50–80% of patients after potentially curative resection of liver metastases from colorectal cancer (Fowler et al. 1993). This fact strongly suggests the presence of micrometastases not visible by diagnostic techniques or during surgical exploration. A number of systemic or local adjuvant chemotherapies have been tested (Fielding et al. 1992), but most results and impressions were disap-

Recent Results in Cancer Research, Vol. 147

pointing (Vaughn and Haller 1993), and survival time was not influenced significantly.

Using an isolated perfusion method in one study the liver was supplied with a high concentration of cytotoxic drugs during the perfusion period, and systemic side effects of the drugs were thereby avoided (Aust and Ausman 1960). If the primary cancer is controlled and there are no other sites of known metastatic disease, the use of isolated liver perfusion techniques may be appropriate for treatment of hepatic metastases. Hyperthermia is becoming an important factor in oncologic strategies (Hamazoe et al. 1991) and can be induced in the liver by isolated perfusion, a technique that is complex and expensive (Aigner et al. 1984; Quebbeman et al. 1984).

We have developed a simple method of isolated hyperthermo-chemo-hypoxic liver perfusion that can be performed as a regional adjuvant therapy in combination with hepatic resection. The unique feature of this method is that it can be done without oxygenation. An oxygenator is thus not necessary in the perfusion circuit, and no blood is required in the perfusate. Moreover, during the perfusion hepatic resection can be performed in a bloodless field with the hepatic metastases visible. Its use depends on the normal hepatic tissue being able to tolerate isolated liver perfusion. The rationale for combining hyperthermia, cytostatic agents, and hypoxia is based on data from other studies and general knowledge about the efficacy of the components on tumor cells.

We previously evaluated the influence of hyperthermo-chemo-hypoxic isolated liver perfusion on the liver and other organs experimentally (Horikawa et al. 1994) and in this study applied it to 11 patients with colorectal hepatic metastases. This report describes that clinical experience.

Materials and Methods

This retrospective study examined the clinical records of 11 patients undergoing hyperthermo-chemo-hypoxic isolated liver perfusion in combination with hepatic resection for colorectal hepatic metastases between 1992 and 1995 at Nara Medical University.

Patient Characteristics

There were six women and five men with a mean age of 55 years (range 45–68 years) (Table 1). Informed consent was obtained from all patients. The location of the primary tumor was the colon in six patients, rectum in four patients, and colon and rectum in one patient. The Original Dukes' stage was B in three patients and C in eight patients. Six patients had a single metastasis, three patients had two metastases, one patient had three metastases, and one patient had seven metastases. In all patients the primary cancer was controlled, and there were no other known sites of metastatic disease. The hepa-

Table 1. Patient characteristics

Patient no.	Age (years)/sex	Site of primary lesion	Duke's stage	Resection timing	Drug used	Sites of liver nodules
1	46/F	Colon	C	Synchronous	CDDP	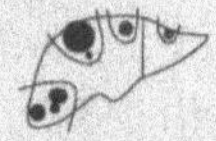
2	56/M	Rectum	C	Synchronous	CDDP	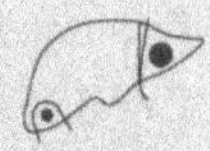
3	59/M	Rectum	C	Synchronous	CDDP	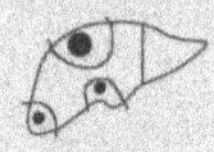
4	51/F	Colon	B	Metachronous	CDDP	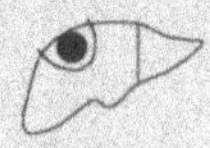
5	68/F	Colon	B	Synchronous	MMC	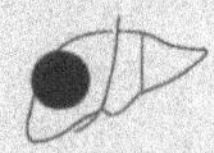
6	68/M	Colon and rectum	B	Metachronous	MMC	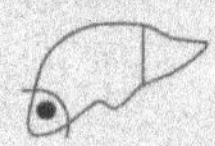
7	50/M	Colon	C	Metachronous	MMC	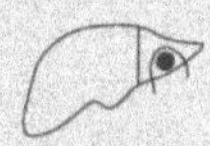
8	53/F	Rectum	C	Synchronous	MMC	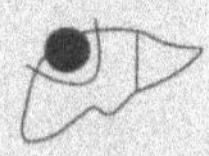
9	58/M	Colon	C	Metachronous	MMC	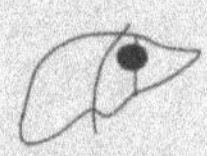
10	54/F	Colon	C	Metachronous	–	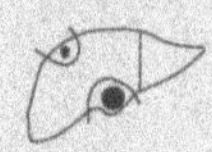
11	45/F	Rectum	C	Synchronous	–	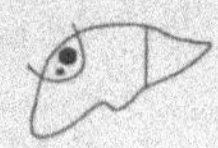

CDDP, cisplatin; *MMC*, mitomycin C

tic resections, which were synchronous in six patients and metachronous in five patients, consisted of eight wedge resections, one left lateral segmentectomy with wedge resection, one right hemihepatectomy, and one left hemihepatectomy.

Hyperthermo-chemo-hypoxic Isolated Liver Perfusion: Technique

Complete dissection of the vascular and ligamentous structures around the liver, especially dissection of the posterior wall of the retrohepatic caval vein and ligation of the right adrenal vein were required to avoid systemic leakage of the perfusate (Fig. 1). After the dissection the portal vein was clamped,

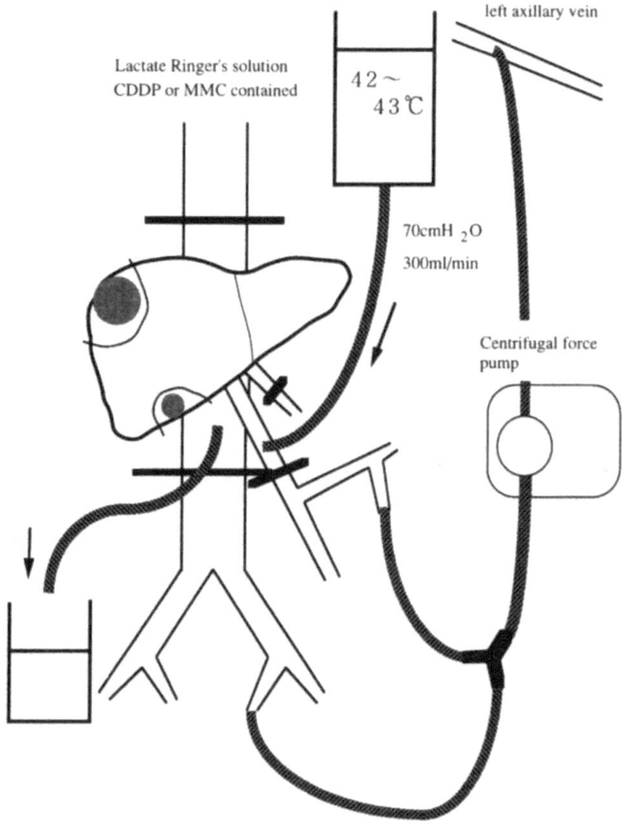

Fig. 1. Hyperthermo-chemo-hypoxic isolated liver perfusion. During isolation of the liver, venovenous bypass was established to stabilize hemodynamic change. *CDDP*, cisplatin; *MMC*, mitomycin C

and a cannula was inserted in the portal vein (the inflow limb for the perfusion). The hepatic artery, infrahepatic caval vein, above the right renal vein, suprahepatic caval vein below the diaphragm, and extrahepatic bile duct were than clamped, in that order; and a cannula was inserted in the caval vein just above the infrahepatic caval clamp (the outflow limb). During isolation of the liver, the venovenous bypass was established so it could return splanchnic and lower systemic venous blood to the axillary vein.

The hepatic perfusion circuit was not closed and did not require a pump-oxygenator. The isolated liver was perfused in vivo for 30 min through a cannula placed in the portal vein by gravity of 70 cm at a rate of approximately 300 ml/min. Lactated Ringer's solution without oxygenation warmed at 42°–43°C was used as the perfusate. The cytotoxic drug mitomycin C (MMC) 10 μg/ml was added to the perfusate in five patients; cisplatin (CDDP) 2 μg/ml was added in four patients; and no cytotoxic drug was used in two patients (Table 1). Hepatic outflow was directed through a cannula placed in the infrahepatic caval vein. During the isolated liver perfusion, hepatectomy was thus performed with a completely bloodless field. After the perfusion the perfusate was washed out, the clamps on the suprahepatic caval vein and hepatic artery were removed, and the hepatic arterial blood inflow was immediately restored. The portal vein and infrahepatic caval vein were then reconstructed.

Clinical Follow-up

The liver temperatures were monitored with a 15-mm needle thermistor probe inserted into the liver during the operation. Samples were obtained from the patients before the start of the perfusion, during the perfusion, 1 h after the perfusion, and daily thereafter to test for glutamic oxaloacetic transaminase (GOT), glutamic pyruvic transaminase (GPT), bilirubin, alkaline phosphatase (ALP), hepaplastin, blood urea nitrogen (BUN), creatinine, and amylase with the use of an autoanalyzer.

Leakage of the cytotoxic drug into the systemic circulation was monitored by bioassay (Fujita 1971) during and after the perfusion.

Patients were followed with monthly laboratory tests (complete blood cell counts, liver function tests, carcinoembryonic antigen analysis). They also underwent a computed tomographic (CT) scan of the abdomen and pelvis and chest radiography every 3 months. Disease recurrence rates were estimated by means of the Kaplan-Meier product limit method.

Results

Changes in Hepatic Tissue Temperature

In 10 of the patients the temperature in the liver reached approximately 40 °C and remained under 42.5 °C during the perfusion (Fig. 2). In patient 9, who died on postoperative day 14 of hepatic failure, it reached 42.9 °C and stayed above 42.5 °C for 20 min. In contrast, body temperature did not change in any of the patients.

Changes in GOT and GPT

The GOT, GPT, and ALP levels were elevated but returned to the normal range within approximately 14 days in most cases (Figs. 3, 4). In patient 9 the GOT and GPT levels were markedly elevated (> 5000 IU and > 3000 IU, respectively). Hepaplastin levels decreased until postoperative day 3 but were restored to normal by postoperative day 7, except in patient 9.

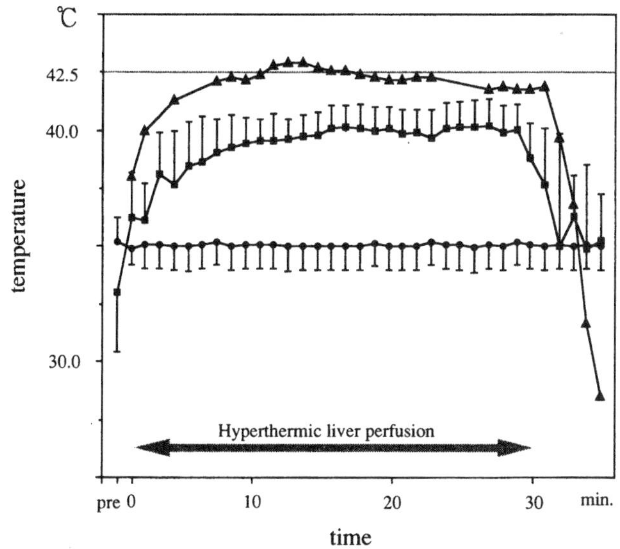

Fig. 2. Changes in hepatic tissue and body temperature of 11 patients undergoing perfusion. ■ Hepatic temperature of 10 patients excluding patient 9; ▲ hepatic temperature of patient 9; ● body temperature of 11 patients. *Vertical bars* indicate mean ± standard deviation

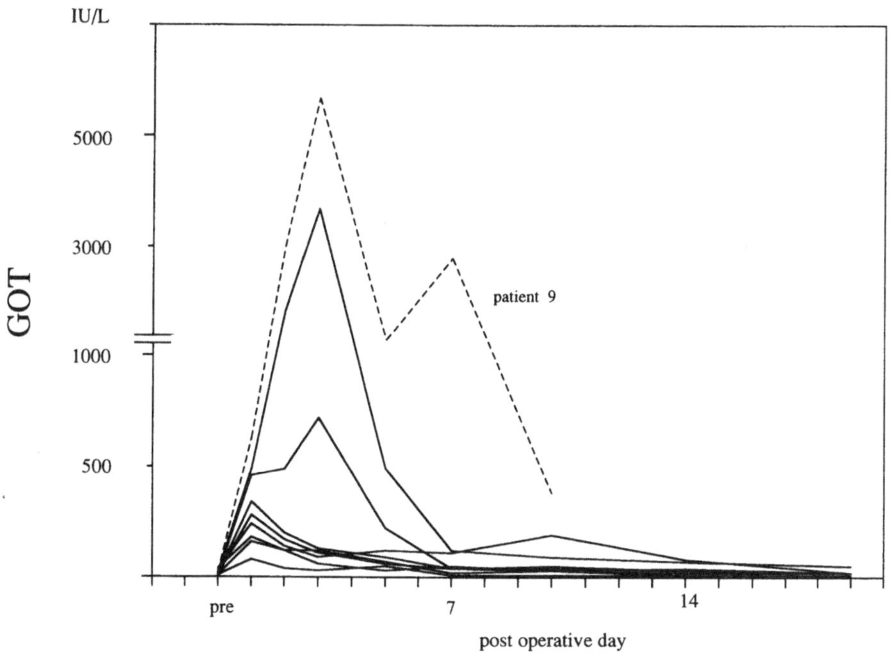

Fig. 3. Changes in glutamic oxaloacetic transaminase (GOT) levels in 11 patients

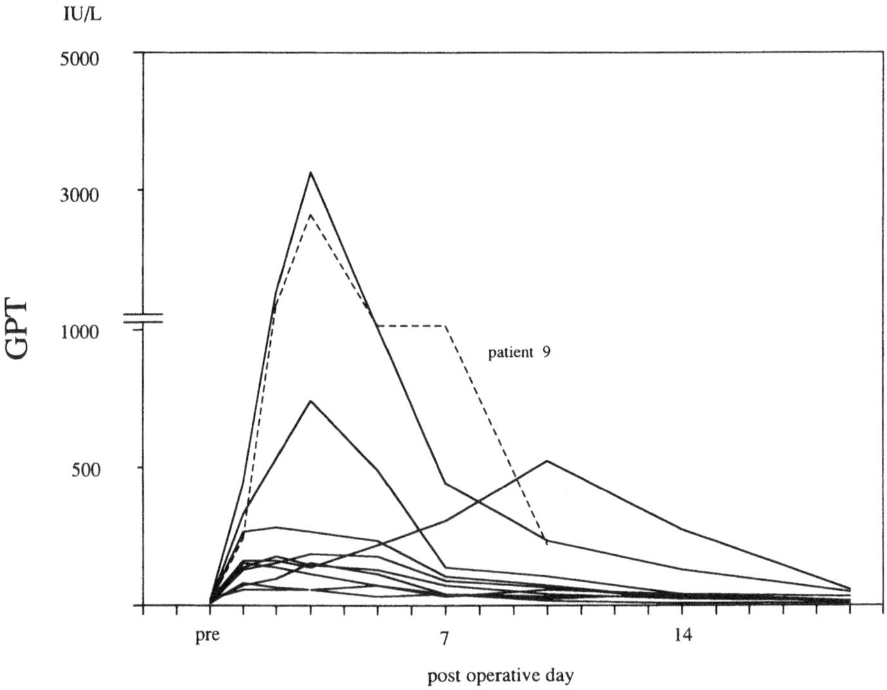

Fig. 4. Changes in glutamic pyruvic transaminase (GPT) levels in 11 patients

Changes in Bilirubin

There were variable transient elevations in the bilirubin level under 5 mg/dl. The elevated levels returned to normal within 14 days, except in patient 9. In patient 9 the bilirubin level was progressively elevated (Fig. 5).

Other Chemical Analyses

In no case was leakage of the cytotoxic drugs into the systemic circulation observed during or after the perfusion. The BUN, creatinine, and amylase levels were not significantly changed after the perfusion, except in patient 9.

Disease Recurrence and Survival

Operative mortality was 9% (1/11). Patient 9, who underwent hyperthermo-chemo-hypoxic liver perfusion using MMC in combination with left hemihepatectomy accounted for the only death. Only in this patient did the temperature in the liver reach 42.5 °C or higher. Morbidity was 18% (2/11: one major problem and one minor one).

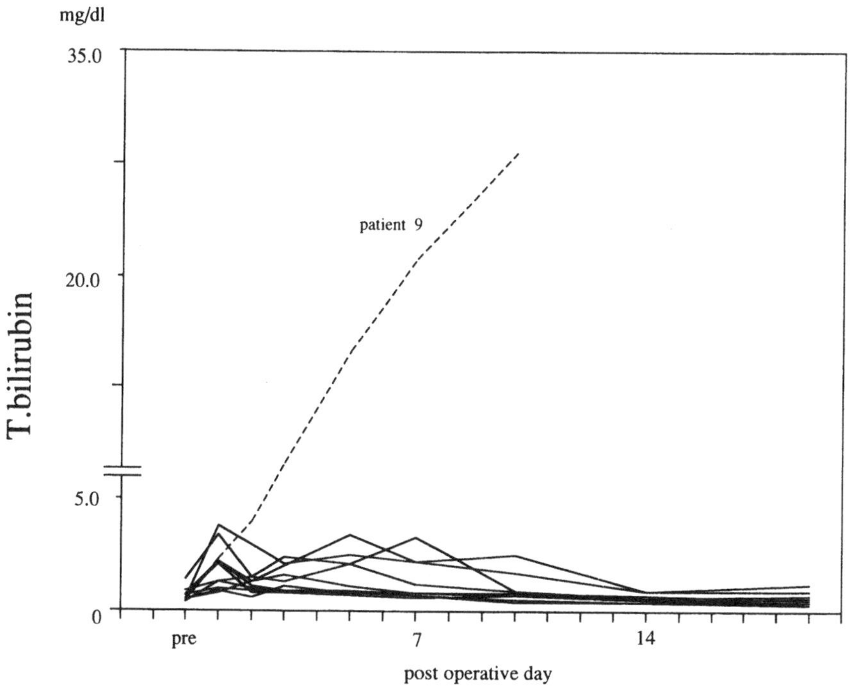

Fig. 5. Changes of total (*T.*) bilirubin levels in 11 patients

Figure 6 shows the results of clinical follow-up of four patients to whom CDDP was administered in the perfusate. Patient 1, who had seven metastases, underwent hyperthermo-chemo-hypoxic isolated liver perfusion in combination with wedge liver resections. Recurrence was found in the liver 19 months after the perfusion. Re-hepatectomy was performed, and the patient died of hepatic recurrence 35 months after the perfusion. Patient 2 had two metastases in both lobes of the liver and underwent left lateral segmentectomy and wedge resection. Bone and lung metastases were found 19 months after the perfusion, and the patient was alive without hepatic recurrence at 27 months. Patient 3 had three metastases, underwent wedge resections, and died of local recurrence 22 months after the perfusion. Patient 4 had a single metastasis, underwent wedge resection, and was alive with no evidence of disease 3 months after the perfusion.

Figure 7 shows the results of clinical follow-up in five patients in whom MMC was administered in the perfusate. Patient 5 had a single, huge metastasis, underwent right hemihepatectomy, and was alive with no evidence of disease 57 months after the perfusion. Patients 6, 7, 8, and 9 had a single metastasis and underwent wedge resection. In patients 6, 7, and 8, extrahepatic recurrences were found at 20, 10, and 7 months, respectively; and they died without intrahepatic recurrence at 24 months (lung and brain), 20 months (bone), and 8 months (lung) respectively, after the perfusion. Patient 9 died on postoperative day 14 owing to hepatic failure.

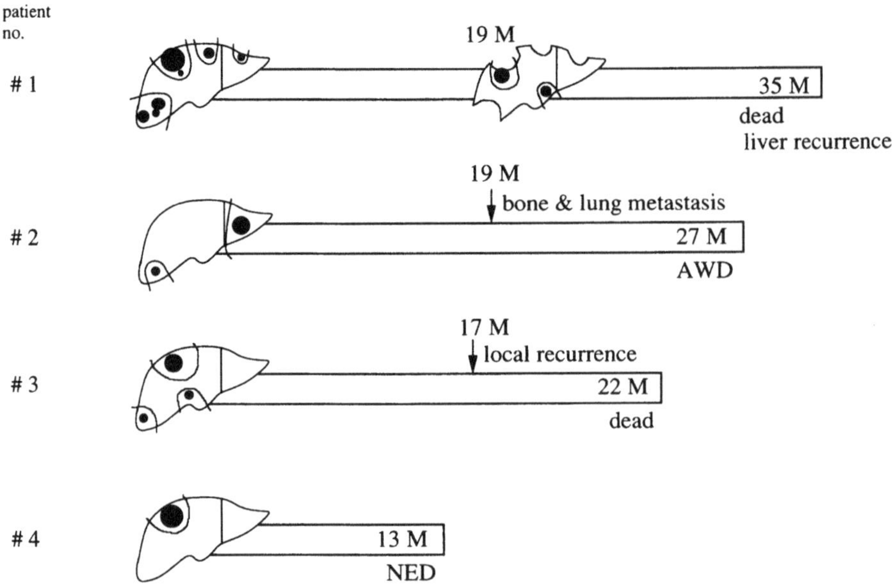

Fig. 6. The results of clinical follow-up for four patients to whom CCDP was administered in the perfusate. *AWD*, Alive with disease; *NED*, no evidence of disease

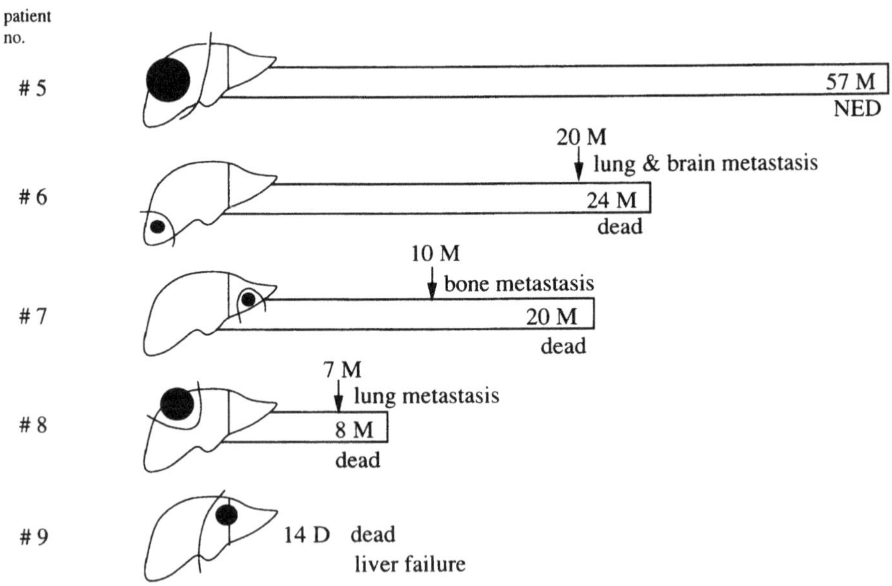

Fig. 7. Results of clinical follow-up for five patients to whom MMC was administered in the perfusate. *D*, days

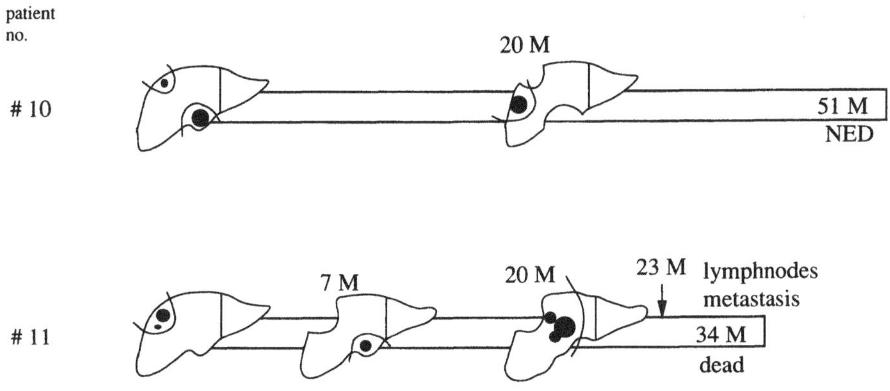

Fig. 8. Results of clinical follow-up for two patients to whom no cytotoxic drugs were administered in perfusate

Figure 8 shows the results of clinical follow-up of two patients to whom no cytotoxic drug was administered in the perfusate. Patient 10 had two metastases in both lobes of the liver and underwent wedge resections. Recurrence in the right lobe was found 20 months after the perfusion. The patient underwent re-hepatectomy and was alive with no evidence of disease 51 months after the perfusion. Patient 11 had two metastases in the right lobe of the liver and underwent wedge resections. Recurrence in the opposite lobe of the liver was found 7 months after the perfusion and the patient underwent re-hepatectomy, but a second hepatic recurrence was found at 20 months. The patient underwent yet another hepatectomy but died of diffuse lymph node metastases at 34 months.

Disease Recurrence Rate

The disease recurrence rate for eight patients who tolerated the perfusion using cytotoxic drugs is shown in Fig. 9. The intrahepatic cumulative recurrence rate was 17% 3 years after the perfusion and the overall recurrence rate was 85%.

Discussion

Liver metastasis from colorectal cancer is a serious problem that must be resolved (Fong et al. 1994). Even with resectable liver metastases, the prognosis is disappointing because of the high rate of postoperative tumor recurrence probably due to residual micrometastases (Fowler et al. 1993). Hepatic resection alone is obviously not adequate treatment, and effective adjuvant modalities are needed for these micrometastatic liver cancers. Such micrometastases may be attributed to the seeding of tumor cells into portal venous

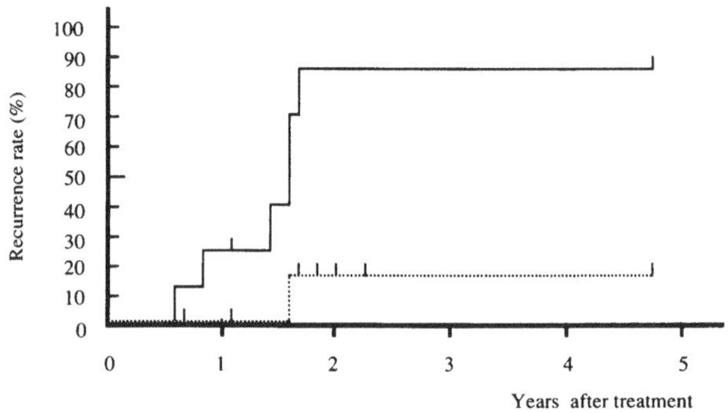

Fig. 9. Disease recurrence rates for eight patients. *Solid line,* overall recurrence rate; *dotted line,* intrahepatic recurrence rate

blood (Taylor et al. 1985), although the blood supply of established visible hepatic metastases is thought to rely entirely on the hepatic artery (Archer and Gray 1990). Therefore regional therapy via the portal vein may be an appropriate treatment of micrometastases.

Effective regional therapy of the liver without inducing systemic damage may be achieved by the isolated liver perfusion technique. Some methods have been described for perfusing the isolated liver via both portal vein and hepatic artery and could be effective even for unresectable hepatic malignancy (Skibba and Quebbeman 1986). The conventional techniques, however, are complicated and expensive because of the need for an extracorporeal circuit with pump-oxygenator and human blood. We developed a simple new system of isolated liver perfusion (hyperthermo-chemo-hypoxic) as a possible adjuvant treatment approach for hepatic metastases. The unique feature of our method is that oxygenation of the perfusate is unnecessary and only the portal vein is used. We need no oxygenator in the system and no blood in the perfusate. Therefore we can carry out liver resection during the perfusion for the visible hepatic metastases with a completely bloodless field. Technically our method closely resembles the method of hypothermic perfused liver resection that was developed to increase resectability in conventionally unresectable hepatic tumors using cold preservation solution as the perfusate (Pichlmayr et al. 1990).

The rationale for combining hyperthermia, a high concentration of cytotoxic agents, and hypoxia against tumor cells is based on data from other studies and general knowledge (Giovanelli et al. 1976; Pigliucci et al. 1993). Before our technique was applied in the clinic, experimental evaluation of its influence on the liver and other organs was required. In our previous experimental study using dogs (Horikawa et al. 1994), the hepatotoxic effect was mild and reversible without systemic toxicity at temperatures in the range of 41 °–42 °C for 30 min, which has a lethal effect on tumor cells even with oxygenation (Radnell et al. 1990).

In the present clinical study we demonstrated the practicability of using hyperthermia, cytotoxic drugs, and ischemia in the human liver in combination with minor or even major hepatic resection. One of the eleven patients died on postoperative day 14 of hepatic failure. The hepatic temperature reached 42.9 °C in this patients, whereas in the other 10 it remained under 42.5 °C. Other reports have shown that a local temperature of 42.5 °C was the upper limit for reversible thermal toxic effect to the human liver (Skibba and Quebbeman 1986). Hence it seems important to control the liver temperature carefully.

Based on the finding that the dose-response relation is steep for MMC, it seems attractive to generate high local drug levels to treat hepatic metastasis (Marinelli et al. 1991). Furthermore, it is well known that hyperthermia accelerates the effect of MMC. The MMC concentration in our perfusate is 10 μg/ml, which is approximately 10 times higher than the clinically achievable peak value in the blood with the conventional mode of administration (Scheithauer et al. 1986). In patients to whom MMC was administered in the perfusate, systemic leakage of the drug was avoided, so there was no sign of systemic toxicity; and no intrahepatic recurrence was observed in our clinical follow-up study (mean 27.3 months, range 8–57 months). Among the four patients for whom CDDP was added to the perfusate at a concentration of 2 μg/ml, intrahepatic recurrence was found in one at follow-up (mean 24.3 months, range 13–35 months). This concentration of the drug – almost the same as the clinically achievable peak value in the blood (Scheithauer et al. 1986) – may be relatively low to avoid hepatic recurrence. Thus for eight patients given cytotoxic drugs in the perfusate, the actuarial intrahepatic recurrence rate was 13% (one of eight) over a mean follow-up of 25.8 months (median 23 months, range 8–57 months), a low incidence compared to the approximately 60% recurrence rate for the historical controls.

In contrast, patients given no cytotoxic drug had hepatic recurrences within 20 months after the perfusion. These findings may indicate the efficacy of and need for cytotoxic drugs in the perfusate of our perfusion system to avoid intrahepatic recurrences.

Although we demonstrated that hyperthermo-chemo-hypoxic isolated liver perfusion could well prevent intrahepatic recurrence, extrahepatic recurrences were often observed. After hepatic resection for colorectal metastases, 25–38% of patients survive a long time without recurrence (Fowler et al. 1993). Hence regional therapy using isolated liver perfusion is not required for these patients. Fifty to eighty percent of patients have subsequent recurrences and in most of these patients there is a possibility not only of intrahepatic but also extrahepatic recurrences. In such cases perfusion may not improve the prognosis. On the other hand, in 21–40% of patients recurrence is limited to the liver, and such a situation is thought to be a potential indication for our intraoperative approach. Unfortunately, absolute criteria have yet to be established for predicting the outcome of hepatic resection (Fong et al. 1994), so in the present study hyperthermo-chemo-hypoxic isolated liver perfusion was applied to all patients with colorectal hepatic metastases. This approach could well avoid intrahepatic, but not extrahepatic, recurrence. Thus establishing selection criteria for this mode of treatment can help us to avoid risks associated with its use.

The present clinical results indicate that hyperthermo-chemo-hypoxic isolated liver perfusion, accomplished with relative ease and low morbidity, is a possible adjuvant treatment in combination with minor or even major hepatic resection in patients with colorectal hepatic metastases. This approach seems effectively to avoid intrahepatic recurrence in properly selected patients, even though there are no absolute criteria for predicting extrahepatic recurrence.

Additional studies are needed to evaluate the limit of the hepatic temperature and dose of the cytotoxic agent in association with the volume of the hepatic resection. Careful clinical follow-up of these patients is required to establish criteria for predicting the likelihood of further recurrence.

References

Aigner KR, Walther H, Tonn JC (1984) Die isolierte Leberperfusion bei fortgeschrittenen Metastasen kolorektaler Karzinome. Onkologie 7:13–21

Archer SG, Gray BN (1990) Comparison of portal vein chemotherapy with hepatic artery chemotherapy in the treatment of liver micrometastases. Am J Surg 159:325–329

Aust JB, Ausman RK (1960) The technique of liver perfusion. Cancer Chemother Rep 10:23–33

Fielding LP, Hittinger R, Grace RH, Fry JS (1992) Randomised controlled trial of adjuvant chemotherapy by portal-vein perfusion after curative resection for colorectal adenocarcinoma. Lancet 340:502–506

Fong Y, Blumgart LH, Cohen A, Fortner J, Brennan M (1994) Repeat hepatic resections for metastatic colorectal cancer. Ann Surg 220:657–662

Fowler WC, Hoffman JP, Eisenberg BL (1993) Redo hepatic resection for metastatic colorectal carcinoma. World J Surg 17:658–662

Fujita H (1971) Comparative studies on the blood level, tissue distribution, excretion and inactivation of anticancer drugs. Jpn J Clin Oncol 12:151–162

Giovanelli BC, Stehlin JS, Morgan AC (1976) Selective lethal effect of supranormal temperatures on human neoplastic cells. Cancer Res 36:3944–3950

Hamazoe R, Murakami A, Hirooka Y, Maeta M, Kaibara N (1991) A phase II pilot study of the combined application of hyperthermia and intra-hepato-arterial chemotherapy using cisplatinum and 5-fluorouracil. J Surg Oncol 48:127–132

Horikawa M, Nakajima Y, Kido K, Ko S, Ohashi K, Nakano H (1994) Simple method of hyperthermo-chemo-hypoxic isolated liver perfusion for hepatic metastases. World J Surg 18:845–851

Marinelli A, Pons DHA, Vreeken JAC, Nagesser SK, Kuppen PJK, Tjaden UR, van de Velde CJH (1991) High mitomycin C concentration in tumor tissue can be achieved by isolated liver perfusion in rats. Cancer Chemother Pharmacol 28:109–114

Pichlmayr R, Grosse H, Hauss J, Gubernatis G, Lamesch P, Bretschneider HJ (1990) Technique and preliminary results of extracorporeal liver surgery (bench procedure) and of surgery on the in situ perfused liver. Br J Surg 77:21–26

Pigliucci GM, Guidice A, Venditti D, Cervelli V, Casciani CU (1993) Optimization of pre-, intra- and postoperative hyperthermic treatment in inoperable lower bowel and liver tumors. Oncology 50:390–392

Quebbeman EJ, Skibba JL, Petroff RJ Jr (1984) A technique for isolated hyperthermic liver perfusion. J Surg Oncol 27:141–145

Radnell M, Jeppsson B, Bengmark S (1990) A technique for isolated liver perfusion in the rat with survival and results of cytotoxic drug perfusion on liver tumor growth. J Surg Res 49:394–399

Scheithauer W, Clark GM, Salmon SE (1986) Model for estimation of clinically achievable plasma concentrations for investigational anticancer drugs in man. Cancer Treat Rep 70:1379–1392

Skibba JL, Quebbeman EJ (1986) Tumoricidal effects and patient survival after hyperthermic liver perfusion. Arch Surg 121:1266–1270

Taylor I, Machin D, Mullee M, Trotter G, Cooke T, West C (1985) A randomized controlled trial of adjuvant portal vein cytotoxic perfusion in colorectal cancer. Br J Surg 72:359–363

Vaughn DJ, Haller DG (1993) Nonsurgical management of recurrent colorectal cancer. Cancer 71:4278–4292

The Surgical Technique of Isolated Hyperthermic Arterial Liver Perfusion in Humans

K.J. Oldhafer[1], H. Lang[1], S. Nadalin[1], M. Frerker[1], W. Schüttler[1], A. Bornscheuer[2], K.-H. Mahr[2], and R. Pichlmayr† [1]

[1] Medizinische Hochschule Hannover, Klinik für Abdominal- und Transplantationschirurgie, Carl-Neuberg-Strasse 1, D-30625 Hannover, Germany
[2] Medizinische Hochschule Hannover, Zentrum Anästhesiologie, Carl-Neuberg-Strasse 1, D-30625 Hannover, Germany

Abstract

Various techniques of isolated liver perfusions have been described, using hepatic artery or both hepatic artery and portal vein. In this paper the technique of isolated arterial liver perfusion is presented. Twelve patients suffering from non-resectable liver tumors underwent this approach. All of them had been previously unsuccessfully treated by resection or systemic chemotherapy. The liver perfusions were performed without technical problems. No operative death occurred. The mean operating time was 413±29 min. Although the perfusion medium was oxygenated and the absolute anoxic period was shorter than 10 min in all cases the perfused livers showed a marked postoperative increase of liver enzyme levels. Further studies should be aimed at reducing this hepatic injury and simplifying the complex surgical procedure.

Introduction

With the availability of new, attractive chemotherapeutic substances for locoregional tumor treatment, isolated liver perfusion is becoming a promising therapy for patients with non-resectable liver tumors (Eggermont et al. 1996; Fraker et al. 1994; Lejeune et al. 1994). The liver can be perfused either via the hepatic artery, the portal vein or both. Several groups have shown that hepatic neoplasms are mainly supplied by the hepatic artery (Ackermann 1974; Lin et al. 1984). Therefore liver perfusion through the hepatic artery might be advantageous in order to reach more tumor cells. We have favored this approach, using only the hepatic artery for liver perfusion. Application of toxic substances like tumor necrosis factor requires complete vascular isolation of the liver. The surgical procedure, including mobilization and vascular isolation of the liver, is in many ways similar to the technique already known from the hepatectomy procedure in liver transplantation or in ex situ liver resections. This paper describes our technique of isolated arterial liver perfusion in the first 12 cases.

Recent Results in Cancer Research, Vol. 147

Surgical Technique

Figure 1 is a schematic diagram of the complete liver perfusion system. The surgical procedure is described step-by-step:

1. Laparotomy and exploration of the abdominal cavity were carried out to confirm, the unresectability of the hepatic malignancy and to exclude extrahepatic tumor growth.
2. The femoral vein and axillary vein were exposed and prepared for insertion of the veno-venous bypass cannulas. The extracorporeal circulation was set up with a centrifugal pump (bio pump, Medtronic-biomedicus, Eden Prairie, Minn. 55344).
3. The hepatoduodenal ligament was divided. Proper and common hepatic arteries were dissected. The gastroduodenal artery was identified and prepared for cannulation. In case of anatomic variations an alternative arterial vessel was used (e.g., the splenic artery; see Table 1)
4. The common bile duct was identified and a prophylactic cholecystectomy performed. The cystic duct was cannulated with a small catheter for collection of bile during the isolated perfusion for pharmacokinetic studies.
5. The portal vein was dissected and prepared for cannulation with the veno-venous bypass cannula.
6. The subhepatic inferior vena cava (IVC) was exposed from the renal veins to the first lower liver veins. In order to obtain enough space for IVC cannulation small lower liver veins were ligated and divided.

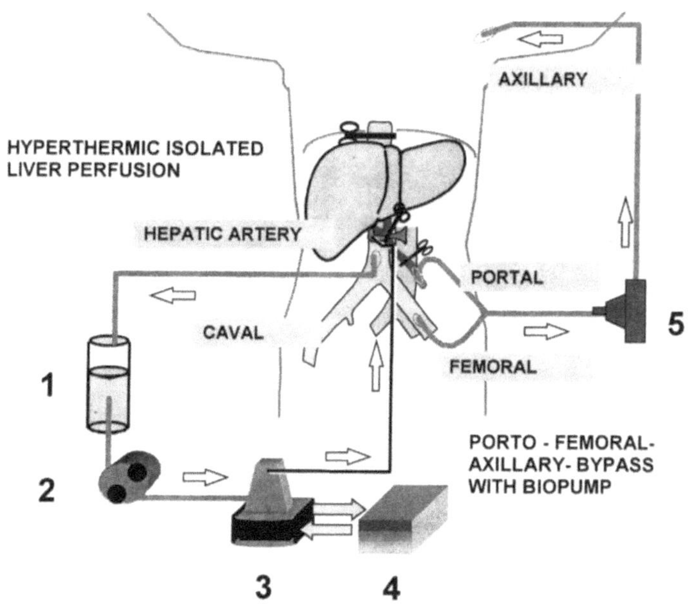

Fig. 1. Schematic diagram of the liver perfusion system: *(1)* venous reservoir; *(2)* roller pump; *(3)* oxygenator; *(4)* heater and *(5)* centrifugal pump

7. The right liver lobe and the retrohepatic vena cava were isolated from the posterior wall of the liver. The right suprarenal vein was divided and ligated (Fig. 2). Thus, complete control of the vena cava was obtained.
8. The suprahepatic IVC was exposed. Phrenic veins were ligated when necessary for clamping of the vena cava without compromising hepatic venous drainage.
9. The sequence of cannulation and clamping was:
   - The gastroduodenal artery was distally ligated, proximally cannulated (Arterial Cannula Pediatric DLP, 10 Fr, Type 77010), and connected with the arterial line of the extracorporeal circuit.
   - The portal (Venous Return Catheter Polystan, 32 Fr, ref. 610032), femoral (Gott-Aneurisma Shunt argyle, 9 mm, ref. 8888-551010) and axillary (Gott-Aneurisma Shunt argyle, 9 mm, ref. 8888-551036) veins were cannulated for veno-venous bypass and bypass perfusion was started.
   - Clamping of the distal part of the subhepatic IVC and cannulation of the proximal part of the IVC were carried out with the venous return cannula through a short cross-incision (Venous Return Catheter Polystan, 32 Fr, ref. 610032; see Fig.3).

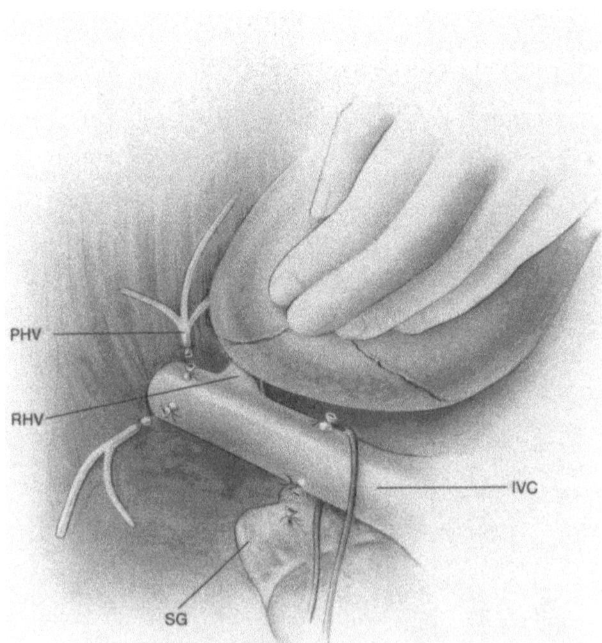

Fig. 2. Mobilization of the right liver lobe. The retrohepatic inverior vena cava is exposed; the suprarenal veins have been divided and ligated. (*SG,* Suprarenal gland; *PHV,* phrenic veins; *RHV,* right hepatic vein)

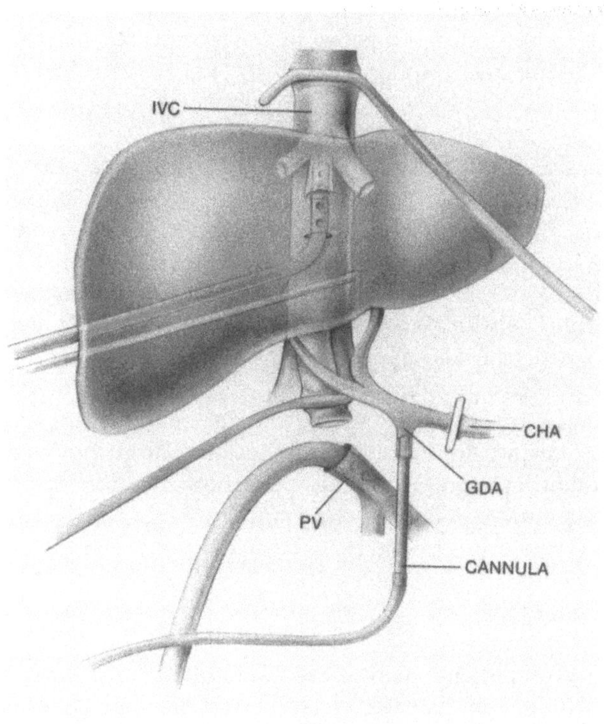

Fig. 3. Operation sites during isolated arterial liver perfusion. (*CHA*, common hepatic artery; GDA, Gastroduodenal Artery; *PV*, portal vein; *IVC*, inferior vena cava)

- The common hepatic artery and suprahepatic IVC were clamped and the isolated liver perfusion was started. Figure 3 shows the sites of operation during isolated liver perfusion.

10. After isolated perfusion wash-out of the liver was performed with 1500 ml saline and 300 ml albumin solution via the arterial cannula and via the portal vein.
11. The common hepatic artery was declamped and arterial reperfusion started; 200–300 ml blood were drained off. Then the suprahepatic IVC was opened.
12. The arterial cannula was withdrawn and the arterial stump of the gastroduodenal artery ligated. As an alternative, an arterial port catheter could be inserted into the stump and fixed.
13. The venous return cannula was removed and the incision closed by running 6–0 Prolene suture.
14. The distal IVC clamp was removed.
15. The portal vein cannula was removed and the portal vein reanastomosed (6–0 Prolene). Portal venous reperfusion was started.
16. Femoral and axillary cannulas were removed and venous incisions closed.

17. The abdomen was temporarily closed.
18. A second-look operation was performed the next day with definitive closure of the abdomen.

Extracorporeal Circuit and Heart-Lung Machine

The extracorporeal circuit consisted of a Hollow Fiber Oxygenator with integrated heat exchanger (Minimax, Medtronic Cardiopulmonary, Anaheim, Calif. 92807) and a computer-aided perfusion system with roller pump and heater (CAPS, Stöckert Instrumente, 80939 Munich, Germany). It was preloaded with 500 ml saline, 250 ml packed red cells and 2000 to 5000 IU heparin. Perfusion flows were adjusted from 400 to 700 ml/min to maintain perfusion pressure below 160 mmHg. Temperature monitoring probes were inserted into the liver and connected with a temperature monitor system. The inflow temperature of the perfusion medium was elevated to 41.0 °C. Perfusion time was limited to 60 min.

Results

Twelve patients with non-resectable liver metastases were treated by this technique of isolated arterial hyperthermic liver perfusion. Patients' diagnoses are shown in Table 1. The operating time was 414±29 min and the anhepatic time was 115±14 min (Table 1). The gastroduodenal artery was used in seven patients for arterial cannulation. In five patients arterial variations were found. In these patients the arterial cannula was inserted into the splenic artery (two patients), common hepatic artery (one patient) and right gastric artery (one patient; see Table 1). The arterial flow varied between 400 and 700 ml/min. In one patient the perfusion was performed via an 8-Fr angiography catheter which was placed in the proper hepatic artery. In this patient a flow of only 250–300 ml/min was possible because of the small inner diameter of 2.2 mm. The veno-venous bypass was performed without problems in all patients. The intestine was well perfused without signs of venous congestion. No operative death occurred and none of the patients suffered postoperative liver failure. In the first postoperative days liver enzyme levels were increased, but almost normalized within 7 days. Figure 3 shows the serum aspartate transaminase levels in the first 10 postoperative days.

Discussion

Isolated arterial liver perfusion represents a complex surgical procedure. The mean operating time was longer than 6 h. However, most steps of this procedure are similiar to the vascular isolation and standardized hepatectomy during liver transplantation. In our hands the surgical technique of isolated arte-

Table 1. Characteristics of patients and operations

Case	Age (years)	Primary tumor	Arterial cannulation	Liver temperature	Operation time (min)	Anhepatic time[a] (min)
1	67	Uveal melanoma	Gastroduodenal artery	41.0 °C	450	102
2	41	Colon cancer	Splenic artery	40.0 °C	410	114
3	49	Colon cancer	Common hepatic artery	40.8 °C	425	89
4	38	Breast cancer	Gastroduodenal artery	41.0 °C	440	110
5	47	Colon cancer	Gastroduodenal artery	40.0 °C	440	107
6	38	Breast cancer	Gastroduodenal artery	41.0 °C	395	120
7	53	Breast cancer	Gastroduodenal artery	40.5 °C	350	120
8	38	Colon cancer	Gastroduodenal artery	40.0 °C	410	116
9	40	Colon cancer	Splenic artery	40.5 °C	420	140
10	48	Colon cancer	Right gastric artery	41.0 °C	435	136
11	39	Small bowel carcinoid	Proper hepatic artery by angiography catheter	36.0 °C	413	115
12	35	Uveal melanoma	Gastroduodenal artery	40.5 °C	375	114

[a] Time from occlusion of the portal vein to portal venous reperfusion.

rial liver perfusion as described above proved to be safe. The occlusion of the suprahepatic IVC without compromising the hepatic venous drainage was very important for the functioning of the extracorporeal perfusion. For this purpose the dissection and clamping of the intradiaphragmatic part of the IVC was helpful. The vascular isolation of the IVC might be troublesome when tumor spread is next to this part of the IVC. Besides drainage of hepatic venous outflow, arterial inflow is another crucial aspect of isolated liver perfusion. The size of the arterial perfusion cannula is very important. The minimum size of the arterial cannula should be 10 Fr to obtain an adequate flow rate.

Whether or not veno-venous bypass is necessary in this procedure remains an open question. We used the bypass for safety reasons. First, it could not be excluded that the patient may not tolerate cross-clamping of the subhepatic IVC and the portal vein as it is practised in conventional liver resection. Second, hyperthermia and the high concentration of chemotherapeutic substances may alter the hepatic tolerance of mesenteric venous congestion and reperfusion. Neither of these events was observed in this series using veno-venous bypass. The veno-venous bypass is, on the other hand, associated with longer operating times and longer anhepatic periods owing to the need for cannulation and de-cannulation of the portal vein and its reconstruction. It could be speculated that in our series, with a perfusion time of 1 h and a wash-out time of 5–10 min, the veno-venous bypass could have been avoided. An alternative might

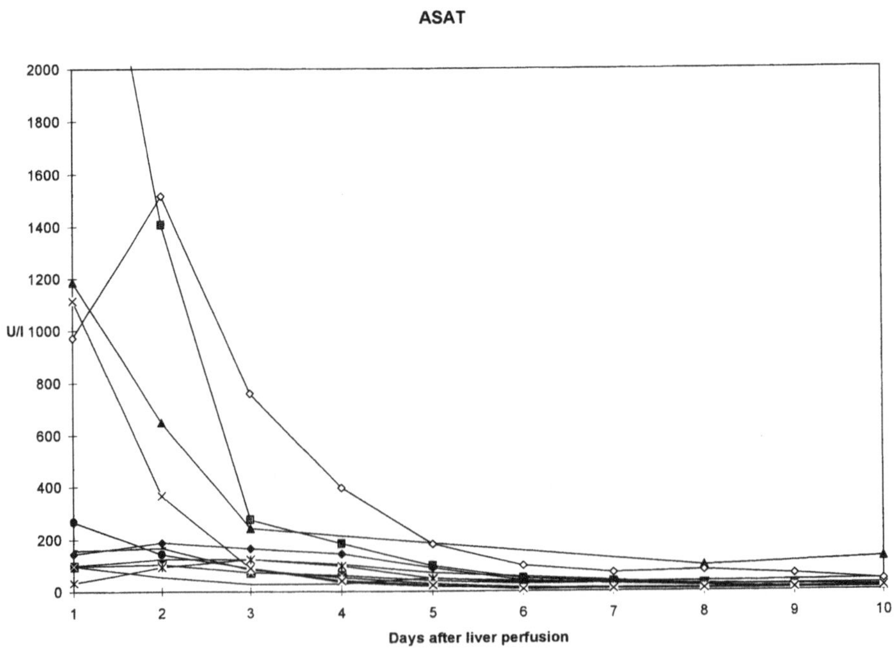

Fig. 4. Serum aspartate transaminase *(ASAT)* concentrations up to 10 days after isolated arterial liver perfusion

be to use the inferior mesenteric vein for cannulation of the porto-mesenteric venous system (Slooff et al. 1989). With this approach portal venous reperfusion can be achieved soon after isolated liver perfusion. Aigner and co-workers have described an intravascular IVC shunt which drained portal and the distal caval veins (Aigner et al. 1982). Cannulation of the femoral and axillary veins could have been avoided by this method, but this shunt appeared to be very complex and had not been applied by many other groups. Generally, when implementation of a longer isolated artificial liver perfusion time is considered in order to increase the tumor killing effect, a veno-venous bypass becomes mandatory.

Although the perfusion medium was oxygenated and the absolute anoxic period was shorter than 10 min in all cases, the perfused livers showed a marked postoperative increase of liver enzymes. The parenchymal damage could be caused by hyperthermia, chemotherapy or artificial perfusion with activation of circulating leukocytes in the extracorporeal circuit. However, it cannot be determined, on the basis of this data, which of these factors was the most important underlying mechanism. In order to minimize this injury, perfusion parameters (flow rate, perfusion pressure, biochemical and hematologic parameters in the perfusion medium) were kept as physiologic as possible. However, efficacy of isolated liver perfusion might be increased by modulating those parameters [e.g., anoxic conditions (Horikawa et al. 1994)]. On the other hand, the liver damage might be aggravated. Perfusion additives may be found capable of reducing hyperthermic and chemotherapeutic toxicity in normal liver cells (Lejeune et al. 1994). The experience gained from research into ischemic/reperfusion injury may also be applied for this modality (Marubayashi and Dohi 1996; Milroy et al. 1995). Substances like oxygen radical scavengers or protease inhibitors may be indicated (Harbrecht et al. 1993).

Reduction of hepatic injury and the simplification of the complex surgical procedure should be key issues of further studies to make isolated liver perfusion more attractive for routine clinical use.

References

Ackermann NB (1974) The blood supply of experimental liver metastases. IV. Changes in vascularity with increasing tumor growth. Surgery 75:589–596

Aigner K, Walther H, Tonn JC, Krahl M, Wenzl A, Merker G, Schwemmle K (1982) Die isolierte Leberperfusion mit 5-Fluorouracil (5-FU) beim Menschen. Chirurg 53:571–573

Eggermont AMM, Koops HS, Klausner JM, Kroon BBR, Schlag PM, Liénard D et al. (1996) Isolated limb perfusion with tumor necrosis factor and melphalan for limb salvage in 186 patients with locally advanced soft tissue extremity sarcomas. Ann Surg 224:756–765

Fraker DL, Alexander HR, Thom AK (1994) Use of tumor necrosis factor in isolated hepatic perfusion. Circ Shock 44:45–50

Harbrecht BG, Billiar TR, Curran RD, Stadler J, Simmons RL (1993) Hepatocyte injury is mediated by proteases. Ann Surg 218:120–128

Horikawa M, Nakajima Y, Kido K, Ko S, Ohashi K, Nakano H (1994) Simple method of hyperthermo-chemo-hypoxic isolated liver perfusion for hepatic metastases. World J Surg 18:845–851

Lejeune FJ, Liénard D, Eggermont AMN, et al. (1994) Clinical experience with high-dose tumor necrosis factor alpha in regional therapy of advanced melanoma. Circ Shock 43:191–197

Lin G, Lunderquist A, Hägerstrand I, Boijsen E (1984) Postmortem examination of the blood supply and vascular pattern of small liver metastases in man. Surgery 96:517–526

Marubayashi S, Dohi K (1996) Therapeutic modulation of free radical-mediated reperfusion injury of the liver and its surgical implications. Surg Today 26:573–580

Milroy SJ, Cottam S, Tan KC, Hilmi I, Oyesola B (1995) Improved haemodynamic stability with administration of aprotinin during orthotopic liver transplantation. Br J Anaesth 5:747–751

Slooff MJH, Bams JL, Sluiter WJ, Klompmaker IJ, Hesselink EJ, Verwer R (1989) A modified cannulation technique for veno-venous bypass during orthotopic liver transplantation. Transplant Proc 21:2328–2329

Monitoring Leakage During Isolated Hepatic Perfusion

P. Lindnér

Department of Surgery, Sahlgrenska University Hospital, Göteborg University, S-413 45 Göteborg, Sweden

Abstract

The toxicity of the drugs used during isolated hepatic perfusion, such as tumor necrosis factor α, necessitates the assessment of leakage. The liver is an organ that, apart from the vessels and the bile duct, can be separated completely from the surrounding body tissue. Leakage can still occur, however, with possible sites at the veins connecting to the caval vein. The caval vein should be freed as much as possible. Drug levels in the perfusate and venous blood can be determined only retrospectively; and because they can be interpreted in different ways they are not sufficient for measuring leakage. If radiolabeled albumin is injected into the perfusion circuit and a detector is placed over the centrifugal perfusion pump (used for the venovenous bypass over the blood reservoir) the accumulation in the systemic blood can be measured. Of all the methods used today this technique seems to be the most sensitive.

Introduction

When isolated limb perfusions were performed more than 30 years ago there was already a need for monitoring leakage. The first paper dealing with the issue was by Stehlin et al. (1961). Iodine-131-labeled human serum albumin (HSA) was used to measure leakage during isolated limb perfusion. Leakage was excessive, but because the drug levels were still fairly low leakage of more than 50% was acceptable. This situation is in contrast to that seem with hepatic or limb perfusion today, where high doses of tumor necrosis factor α (TNFα) are used and the dose given to the perfused organ is sometimes as much as 10 times higher than the highest tolerable systemic dose. Therefore leakage must be less than 10%.

During isolated hepatic perfusion (IHP) it is necessary in addition to assessing leakage, to monitor and record the temperature, blood pressure, and blood flow in the perfusion circuit. Today these measurements can be easily attained with a personal computer or Macintosh-based system that displays

Recent Results in Cancer Research, Vol. 147

the leakage rate and other physiological parameters in real time for the surgeon in a practical manner.

Possible Leakage Routes

In contrast to the limbs, the liver is an organ that, except for the vessels and the bile duct, can be freed completely from the surrounding body tissue. Leakage should therefore be a minor problem during IHP. When leakage does occur, however, where does the fluid go? If the caval vein is not freed at the rear, leakage via veins connecting to the caval vein is possible. Leakage can also occur via veins from the diaphragm. The technique for isolating the caval vein is of great importance. In Göteborg we first adopted the technique of Aigner et al. (1983), isolating the suprahepatic caval vein at the level of the pericardium. More recently we have used a technique that resembles the hepatectomy performed during liver transplantation: The caval vein is separated completely at the rear. If the liver is greatly enlarged, this procedure can be difficult to perform, reducing isolation only to above and below the liver. Leakage may also occur via lymph vessels from the liver. Thirty percent of the lymph flow in the thoracic duct originates from the liver. All structures attached to the liver are therefore carefully divided during the separation. A possible means of leakage during IHP is the bleeding, or "sweating," that occurs during perfusion. This fluid may be reabsorbed from the peritoneal cavity if it is not suctioned out.

Indirect Measurement of Leakage

By measuring and comparing the drug levels in the perfusate and the venous blood it is possible to demonstrate the concentration gradient between the perfusion circuit and the systemic blood. In Fig. 1 the level of cisplatin in the perfusate is shown to be as much as 100 times higher than the cisplatin concentration in the systemic blood (Naredi et al. 1992). As the cisplatin concentration decreases in the perfusion circuit it may denote leakage; it may also be explained by an increase in the amount of cisplatin entering the liver cells or an increase in protein binding over time. As these measurements can be made only retrospectively and can be interpreted in various ways, they are insufficient for measuring leakage.

The results are clearer if a radioactive tracer is injected into the perfusion circuit, and systemic blood samples are obtained. Figure 2 shows how the concentration of tracer in the liver decreases and the content of tracer in the wound increases, which can be explained by bleeding from the liver. Assays on such blood samples cannot replace direct measurements but are necessary to validate the accuracy of a real-time measurement.

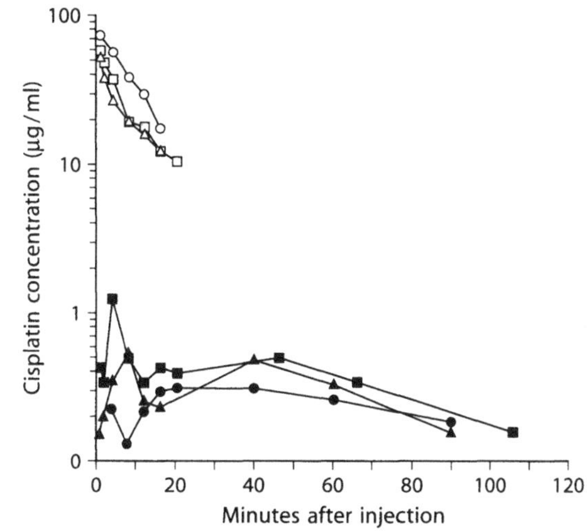

Fig. 1. Time course of cisplatin in the perfusion circuit (open symbols;) and plasma (closed symbols;) in three patients during regional hyperthermic cisplatin perfusion (From Naredi et al. 1992, with permission)

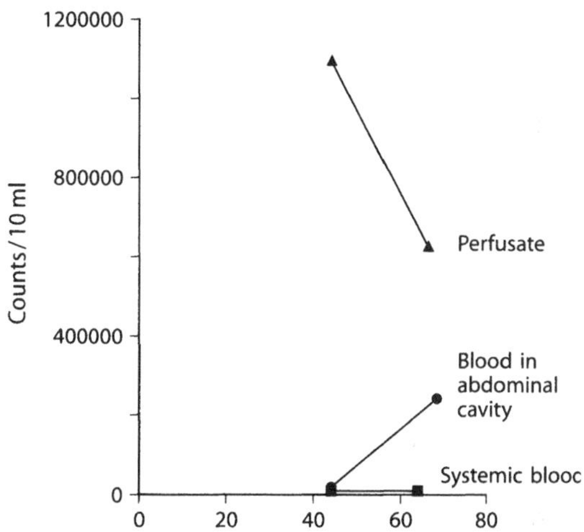

Fig. 2. Technetium-99 labeled erythrocytes injected into the liver perfusion circuit. Samples from the perfusate, blood, and abdominal cavity, were obtained 20 min later

Direct Measurement of Leakage

In 1987 a group from Leiden (Runia et al. 1987) presented a study of continuous measurements of leakage during isolated liver perfusion in pigs. They used Technetium-99-labeled erythrocytes injected into the perfusion circuit. In their first experiments they placed the detector over the heart, but after problems with reproducibility the system was changed and the detector was placed over an arteriovenous shunt. Two examples are depicted in Fig. 3: one case with leakage and one without.

The best system for measuring leakage was described by Barker et al. (1995). In their system a small amount of iodine-131-labeled HSA is injected

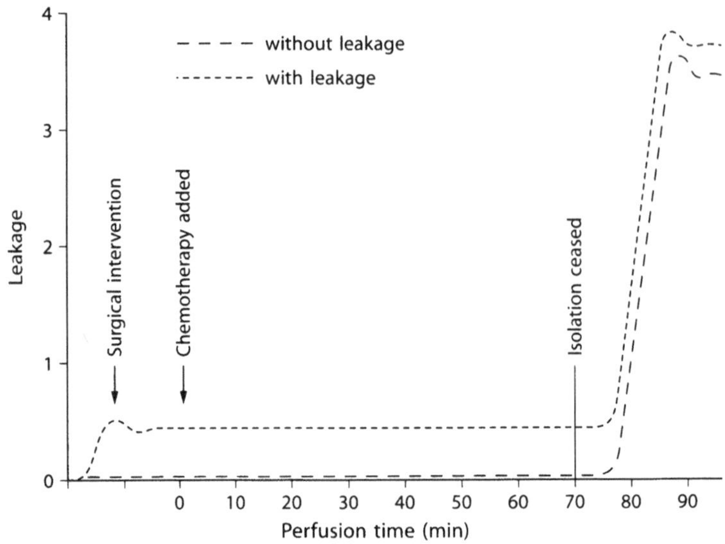

Fig. 3. Representative leakage measurements during the course of perfusion with and without leakage (From Runia et al. 1987, with permission)

into the systemic circulation to establish a baseline count, correcting for background radiation. After waiting 5–10 min for stabilization, 10 times the amount of radiolabeled albumin (400 μCi) is injected into the perfusion circuit. The detector is then placed over the centrifugal perfusion pump used for the venovenous bypass over the blood reservoir.

At our instituion, leakage is demonstrated by calculating the disappearance rate from the perfusion circuit. Technetium-labeled erythrocytes are injected into the perfusion circuit, and the detector is placed over the liver during perfusion. In the five patients subjected to this technique, leakage has been between 5% and 25% per hour. The leakage rate of one patient is depicted in Fig. 4.

Discussion

Problems arise when leakage is monitored by calculating the disappearance rate of the tracer from the liver. This technique requires the detector situated over the liver which can create operational difficulties; moreover, it may become necessary to remove the detector if surgical correction is needed. Another disadvantage is that the disappearance of isotope can be explained in different ways. It may indeed be true leakage into the systemic circulation, but it may also be due to bleeding, where radioactivity leaks into the abdominal cavity and must suctioned out.

The advantages with the system used at the U.S. National Institutes of Health (Barker et al. 1995) are that the detector is placed at a distance from the sterile operating area, and the system has high sensitivity (< 1%). A pos-

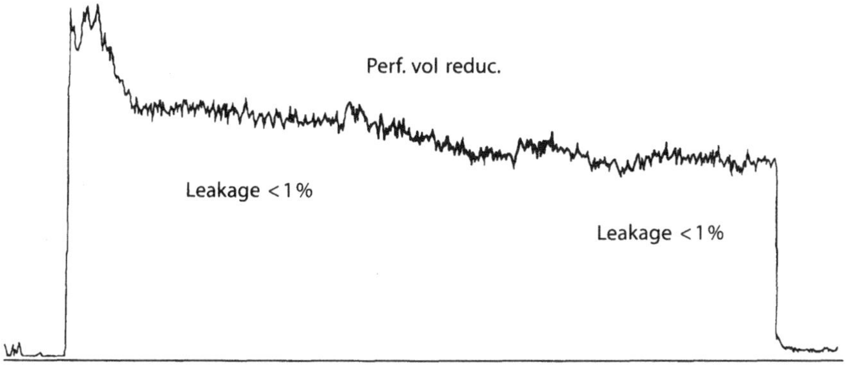

Fig. 4. Patient 2. A leakage rate of >1% per 10 min was calculated from erythrocyte technetium-99-studies that suddenly increased. At inspection there was bleeding from the portal vein where the catheter entered the vessel. When the catheter was adjusted, leakage decreased to the previous level

sible problem with a system that measures accumulation in the systemic circulation is that there may be tracer in the reticuloendothelial system in the liver, which could cause the amount of leakage to be underestimated. Hence a tracer stable in the systemic circulation must be used, such as radiolabeled HSA, which has a half-life of approximately 7 h.

In conclusion, to avoid leakage during liver perfusion and especially leakage from the caval vein, the vein should be freed as much as possible. A real-time monitoring system should be used to determine the volume of the leakage. Finally, it is advantageous to place the detector over the systemic circulation (e.g., over the pump to the venovenous bypass).

References

Aigner K, Walther H, Tonn J, Wénzl A, Hechtel R, Merker G, Schwemmle K (1983) First experimental and clinical results of isolated liver perfusion with cytotoxics in metastases from colorectal primary. Cancer Res 86:99–102

Barker WC, Andrich MP, Alexander HR, Fraker DL (1995) Continuous intraoperative external monitoring of perfusate leak using iodine-131 human serum albumin. Eur J Nucl Med 22:1242–1248

Naredi P, Holmberg SB, Hafström L, Heath DD, Shalinsky DR, Howell SB (1992) Pharmacokinetics of cisplatin in an isolated liver perfusion system in humans. Reg Cancer Treat 4:254–257

Runia RD, De Brauw LM, Kothuis BJL, Pauwels EKJ, Van De Velde GJH (1987) Continuous measurement of leakage during isolated liver perfusion with a radiotracer. Nucl Med Bio 14:113–118

Stehlin JS, Glark RL, Dewey W (1961) Continuous monitoring of leakage during regional perfusion. Arch Surg 83:165–171

Anesthesiological Management During Isolated Liver Perfusion

A. Bornscheuer, K.H. Mahr, K. Kirchhoff, K.J. Oldhafer, H. Lang, and S. Piepenbrock

Zentrum Anästhesie, Abteilung I, Medizinische Hochschule Hannover, Carl-Neuberg-Strasse 1, D-30625 Hannover, Germany

Abstract

The treatment of irresectable hepatic metastases is limited by the systemic toxicity of anticancer agents. Isolated hyperthermic liver perfusion (IHLP) with anticancer agents is a new therapy for irresectable liver tumors. The risks of this therapy lie in the extended operation, the anhepatic phase and the possibility of liver damage due to the anticancer drugs and hyperthermia. Experience of this method is rare, and the side effects are not well known. To estimate the individual risk of patients before isolated liver perfusion an extended evaluation of the preoperative conditions is usual. Titration of all anesthetic agents is advisable to prevent cardiovascular changes and to avoid an extended recovery time after therapy. Based on our experience with IHLP in ten patients, we prefer coinduction with midazolam and thiopentone. After intubation, intermittent positive pressure ventilation with positive end-expiratory pressure is instituted with 30% oxygen in air. Pancuronium bromide is used to provide muscular paralysis, and isoflurane is administered throughout the procedure. Anesthesia is supplemented by fentanyl and midazolam.

Invasive hemodynamic monitors may be placed after induction of anesthesia.

Our first results with IHLP indicate that, under the conditions of elevated monitoring, complete isolation of the liver, a good wash-out and a safe anesthesiological management, no major disturbances must be expected during the therapy. The patients are more compromised by the therapy during the following days. Low diastolic blood pressure and loss of resistance after perfusion were the first signs of a toxic reaction.

Introduction

The treatment of irresectable hepatic metastases is limited by the systemic toxicity of anticancer agents. Isolated hyperthermic liver perfusion (IHLP) with anticancer agents is a new therapy for irresectable liver tumors, which has been used in only a few centers so far (Aigner et al. 1984; Hafström et al.

Recent Results in Cancer Research, Vol. 147

1994; Quebbeman et al. 1984). The benefits of IHLP are high local concentration of antitumor agents with maximization of antitumor efficacy and reduction of systemic side effects. The risks of this therapy lie in the extended operation, the anhepatic phase and the possibility of liver damage due to the anticancer drugs and hyperthermia. The risk of anoxic liver damage can be excluded by using a heart-lung machine as a perfusate oxygenator. After unsatisfactory systemic cytostatic therapy IHLP is an alternative in the treatment of irresectable hepatic tumors.

The perioperative care of patients undergoing isolated liver perfusion is one of the most challenging clinical situations that the surgeon and anesthesiologist currently encounter. Experience of this method is rare and the side effects are not well known. This therapy is associated with the risk of various complications. The surgical technique is very difficult and requires great surgical experience (venovenous bypass, heart-lung machine, liver isolation). The changes during perfusion are similar to the changes during the anhepatic phase in orthotopic liver transplantation (coagulation disorders, imbalances in the acid-base and electrolyte metabolism, hypoglycemia, renal failure). Complete isolation of the liver must be guaranteed to prevent systemic leakage of the perfusate. The reperfusion period can be complicated by the inflow of toxic metabolites and anticancer agents from the perfused liver into the organism. The most frequent complication after mitomycin C perfusion is veno-occlusive disease (Craft and Pembrey 1987; Takayasu et al. 1990; Verweij and Stoter 1987). After cisplatin and melphalan perfusion it is activation of the coagulation system (Arnestad et al. 1992). The condition of the patients can be reduced by side effects of previous systemic anticancer therapy, thus, there is obvious necessity of careful perioperative monitoring and anesthesiological management.

Preoperative Assessment

To estimate the individual risk of patients before isolated liver perfusion an extended evaluation of the preoperative conditions is usual. Assessment of the patients should include case history, physical examination, blood pressure, volume state and electrocardiography. In case of arrhythmia or signs of heart disease, an echocardiogram is useful in identifying severe cardiac dysfunctions. Severe heart disease can be a contraindication for this invasive therapy.

Assessment of the patient's pulmonary function includes chest radiography and lung function tests. Analysis of arterial blood gases is not necessary in case of good lung function. The preoperative evaluation also includes renal function tests, electrolyte balance and blood glucose. A complete blood count is made and the coagulation system is checked. The investigation of the coagulation system includes platelet count, Quick's test, partial thromboplastin time (PTT), fibrinogen, prothrombin (FII) and proaccelerin (FV). The determination of fibrin degradation products can be helpful to detect hyperfibrinolysis (history of abdominal operation).

Safety Precautions

Isolated liver perfusion requires safety precautions for the staff. Personnel should be informed about the special risk in association with anticancer agents. Special gloves (thickness 0.25–0.3 mm), glasses and work clothes should be worn. All collected blood samples must be marked as cytostatics contaminated. Contaminated material, blood and urine must be disposed of in separate bins for cytostatic waste.

Anesthesia

Based on our experience in ten patients with IHLP we prefer the following anesthesiological management protocol: in the evening before the operation patients are given a somnific (pentobarbital); 45 min before arrival in the anesthetizing room the patient undergoes premedication with 5–7.5 mg midazolam orally; the patient is positioned on a warming mattress on the operating table with both arms extended laterally; after arrival in the anesthetizing room standard monitoring equipment (electrocardiogram, blood pressure cuff and pulse oximeter) is attached; after insertion of a large canula (14 G) in a peripheral vein 500–1000 ml crystalloids should be given. If the premedication is not satisfactory, we give 1.5–3 mg midazolam intravenously as an anxiolytic and coinduction agent. After preoxygenation and precurarization anesthesia is induced with thiopentone (3–5 mg/kg body weight). After intubation, intermittent positive pressure ventilation with positive end-expiratory pressure (5 mmHg) is instituted with 30% oxygen in air. Ventilation should be adjusted to maintain an end-tidal carbon dioxide concentration between 4,5 and 5%. Pancuronium bromide is used to provide muscular paralysis and isoflurane is administered throughout the procedure. Anesthesia is supplemented by fentanyl and midazolam. Normally the degree of liver dysfunction in patients presenting for isolated liver perfusion is not severe. Therefore, drug disposition in these patients is usually almost normal. During the anhepatic phase the hepatic clearance of drugs ceases and the amount of anesthetic agents needed is reduced. In addition, after isolated liver perfusion, hepatic extraction is influenced by the maximal intrinsic capacity of metabolizing enzymes to clear a drug. Therefore, anesthetic drugs with an enzyme-limited clearance (thiopental, diazepam) should be given very carefully. Titration of all anesthetic agents is advisable to prevent cardiovascular changes and to avoid an extended recovery time after therapy.

Monitoring

Invasive hemodynamic monitors may be placed after induction of anesthesia. A radial artery catheter is inserted to collect blood samples and to measure arterial diastolic (BPdia) and systolic (BPsys) blood pressure. A central venous line (drug therapy) and a second venous canula (volume) are placed. A Swan-Ganz Catheter is inserted via the internal jugular vein. The placement of a pulmonary artery catheter allows continuous monitoring of pulmonary artery (PAP) and central venous (CVP) pressure and intermittent measurement of pulmonary capillary wedge pressure (PCWP) and cardiac output (CO). Mean arterial blood pressure [MAP: BPdia+(BPsys-BPdia)/3], total vascular resistance [PVR: (MAP–CVP)×80/CO] and pulmonary vascular resistance [PVR: (PAP–PCWP)×80/CO] are calculated. Temperature is measured via the Swan-Ganz Catheter and a rectal thermometer. A vesical tube is inserted to measure urinary output. We evaluate coagulation parameters (Quick's test, PTT, fibrinogen, FII and FV) and perform hemanalysis, as well as analyzing electrolytes (sodium, potassium, calcium), lactate, blood sugar and arterial and mixed venous blood gas during therapy. In addition, arteriovenous oxygen difference ($avDO_2$: arterial oxygen content – mixed-venous oxygen content), oxygen consumption (OC: $avDO_2 \times CO$) and intrapulmonary shunt (Qs/Qt: (alveolar oxygen tension – paO_2)×0.031/$avDO_2$+(alveolar oxygen tension – paO_2)×0.0031) are calculated. Measurements are usually made (a) at the beginning of surgery, (b) 10 min before and (c) 10 min after starting isolated perfusion, (d) 10 min before the end of perfusion and (e) 10 and (f) 60 min after reperfusion. These fixed measurements are completed in case of unexpected interruptions.

First Experience

Patients

We performed IHLP in ten patients with isolated irresectable liver tumors. In six cases the anticancer agent in the perfusate was mitomycin and in four cases tumor necrosis factor (TNF) and melphalan. Biometric data and primary tumors of the patients are shown in Table 1. The American Society of Anesthesiologists classification of all patients was stage II. None of the patients had a history of heart or pulmonary disease. One patient had insulin-dependent diabetes and one had hypertension. The general condition of the patients with a history of breast carcinoma, radiation treatment and chemotherapy was reduced. During the operation period CVP should be above 9 mmHg and hemoglobin content above 9 g/dl. The duration of the operation and the required volume during the operation are shown in Table 2.

Hemodynamics

The course of circulation up to reperfusion was similar to the course during orthotopic liver transplantation in tumor patients using a venovenous bypass. At the beginning of the anhepatic period, heart rate increased significantly from 74±10 to 87±12 beats/min ($P<0.05$). The mean blood pressure

Table 1. Biometric data

Patient no.	Primary tumor	Sex	Age (years)	Height (cm)	Weight (kg)
1	Malignant melanoma	Male	67	172	85
2	Sigmoid carcinoma	Female	47	170	65
3	Breast cancer	Female	38	165	65
4	Colon carcinoma	Male	49	180	102
5	Colon carcinoma	Female	41	169	56
6	Breast cancer	Female	38	170	66
7	Breast cancer	Female	43	175	81
8	Sigmoid carcinoma	Female	48	158	74
9	Colon carcinoma	Female	38	164	60
10	Colon carcinoma	Male	40	178	71

Table 2. Operation time, volume substitution and urine production

Patient no.	Operation time (min)	Anhepatic period (min)	Fresh frozen plasma (units)	Packed red blood cells (units)	Crystalloids (ml)	Colloids (ml)	Urine production (ml)
1	450	102	7	6	7500	1000	1200
2	410	114	6	9	4000	500	485
3	425	89	5	2	5500	500	2500
4	440	110	4	6	7000	1000	2400
5	440	107	4	7	6000	1000	2200
6	395	120	6	7	4000	1000	550
7	350	120	0	2	5000	500	1525
8	410	116	6	3	5000	500	3250
9	420	140	6	2	5500	500	3760
10	435	136	7	7	5600	500	2385
11	413	115	6	6	6500	0	1430
12	375	114	8	5	8500	500	3000

(69±8 to 71±10 mmHg) and the CVP (10±4 to 9±4 mmHg) were unchanged by the anhepatic phase. Cardiac output decreased significantly from 6.4±1.2 to 5±1.1 l/min ($P<0.05$), PAP from 21±4.1 to 17±3.7 mmHg ($P<0.05$) and PCWP from 14±3.7 to 10±3.7 mmHg ($P<0.05$); TVR increased significantly from 776±209 to 1068±373 dyn sec cm^{-5} ($P<0.05$). During the reperfusion period the hemodynamic values returned to baseline. No arrhythmias or bradycardias were observed. Within the first hour after reperfusion diastolic blood pressure decreased significantly from 58±11.4 to 46±11.2 mmHg ($P<0.05$) and TVR from 1011±219 to 567±220 dyn sec cm^{-5} ($P<0.05$); CO increased from 5.1±0.9 to 8.2±2.1 l/min ($P<0.05$). At the end of the operation only diastolic blood pressure and TVR were significantly changed in comparison with the beginning [59±7 to 46±11 mmHg and 825±206 to 567±219 dyn sec cm^{-5} ($P\leq0.05$) respectively]. The reperfusion syndrome was more pronounced in patients after TNF application than after mitomycin C application. One of six pa-

Table 3. Hemodynamic measurements mode at the beginning of surgery *(A)*, 10 min before *(B)* and 10 min after *(C)* starting isolated perfusion, 10 min before the end of perfusion *(D)* and 10 min *(E)* and 60 min *(F)* after reperfusion

	A	B	C	D	E	F
Heart rate(beats/min)	73±9*	74±10	87±12*	87±15	90±15	91±12
BPsy (mmHg)	105±14	99±10	102±12	102±10	100±11	102±11
BPdia (mmHg)	59±7	55±7	56±9	58±11	49±9*	46±11
CVP (mmHg)	10±6	10±4	9±4	10±3	10±3	11±3
PAP (mmHg)	21±6	21±4	17±4*	17±4	18±4	21±4
PCWP (mmHg)	13±5	14±4	10±4*	10±3	10±3	12±3*
CO (l/min)	6.5±1.4	6.4±1.2	5.2±1*	5.1±1	6.4±2.3*	8.2±2.1
TVR (dyn sec cm^{-5})	825±206	776±210	1005±332*	1011±219	784±322*	567±219
PVR (dyn sec cm^{-5})	94±39	90±28	104±36	121±36	113±39	91±35

BPsys, Systolic blood pressure; BPdia, diastolic blood pressure; *CVP*, central venous pressure; *PAP*, pulmonary arterial pressure; *PCWP*, pulmonary wedge pressure; *CO*, cardiac output; *TVR*, total vascular resistance; *PVR*, pulmonary vascular resistance.
* = $P < 0.05$.

tients in the mitomycin C group and three of four in the TNF group required vasopressor agents for a short period. During the second-look operation on the next day none of the mitomycin C patients, but two of the TNF patients, needed norepinephrine to elevate MAP. Vasopressor agents were used if MAP was lower than 55 mmHg and did not increase after volume substitution. All results of the hemodynamic measurements are shown in Table 3.

Blood Gas Analysis

In all patients, oxygen uptake and carbon dioxide output were unaffected by the therapy. Only during the anhepatic period did the carbon dioxide levels in the blood gas analysis decrease not significantly from 34.5 ± 2.1 to 32.7 ± 3.9 mmHg and the end-expiratory carbon dioxide concentration decreased significantly from 4.3 ± 0.2 to 3.9 ± 0.4 vol.% ($P < 0.05$). These changes were caused by the isolation of the liver from the organism. Base excess was -1.92 ± 2.71 mmol/l at the beginning of the operation, -4.82 ± 2.82 mmol/l during the therapy, -5.19 ± 2.37 mmol/l after reperfusion and -2.63 ± 1.9 mmol/l at the end of the operation. The changes in base excess during therapy and after reperfusion were significant ($P < 0.05$). The patients required a mean of 125 ± 200 ml sodium bicarbonate solution.

Calculated Oxygen and Circulation Parameters

The $avDO_2$ was not changed at the beginning of the anhepatic period. After reperfusion $avDO_2$ increased significantly from 2.5 ± 0.5 to 3 ± 0.6 ml/100 ml

($P < 0.05$). During the anhepatic period the oxygen consumption was significantly ($P < 0.05$) lower (67 ± 13 and 68 ± 9 ml/min/m^2) than at the beginning of the operation (98 ± 16 ml/min/m^2) and the end of the operation (111 ± 36 ml/min/m^2). The difference between the oxygen consumption at the beginning and at the end of the operation was not significant. The calculated intrapulmonary right-to-left shunt was unchanged during the observation period, due to the excellent isolation of the liver during the hyperthermic perfusion and a complete wash-out after perfusion.

Blood Glucose and Lactate

Three patients were hypoglycemic at the beginning of the operation. They required a glucose infusion to normalize blood sugar levels. The blood sugar levels of all patients decreased significantly during the anhepatic period from 7.1 ± 2.7 to 5.5 ± 1.6 mmol/l ($P < 0.05$). This finding reflects the absence of gluconeogenesis during this period. After reperfusion blood sugar levels increased significantly to 9.6 ± 2.9 mmol/l ($P < 0.05$). Lactate increased significantly from 0.92 ± 0.4 mmol/l at the beginning to 4.3 ± 1.7 mmol/l after reperfusion. During the first hour after reperfusion lactate levels decreased to 3.2 ± 0.66 mmol/l (not significant).

Electrolyte Metabolism

The sodium concentration increased significantly over the whole operation period from 143.1 ± 2.5 to 147 ± 2.2 mmol/l ($P < 0.05$). The reason for this increase was the correction of acidosis with sodium bicarbonate solution. Potassium showed no significant changes. Potassium depletion was treated with 20–40 mVal potassium chloride. No significant changes in calcium metabolism were observed.

Temperature

Central body temperature decreased significantly from 36.1 ± 0.4 to $35.5 \pm 0.4\,^{\circ}$C during the preparation time ($P < 0.05$). Thereafter body temperature remained unchanged.

Hemoglobin and Coagulation System

Hemoglobin was constant during the observation period. The first six patients (mitomycin C) were treated with systemic anticoagulation therapy (heparin: 250 IU/kg body weight) during the hyperthermic perfusion. Coagulation parameters decreased slightly due to hemodilution (crystalloids, colloids). In the anhepatic period changes in the coagulation system were caused by heparinization (elevated PTT, decreased Quick's test, FII and FV values). Bleeding after declamping of the vessels was easily controlled in all patients by surgical hemostasis. Therefore heparin neutralization was not performed except in the first patient. In one patient the coagulation status was limited at the start of operation. This patient showed signs of intravascular coagulation after reperfusion. In the last four patients (TNF, melphalan) no heparinization was performed. No coagulation disorders were observed in this group.

Perfusate

The perfusate consisted of two units packed red blood cells and 400 ml physiological sodium solution. To prevent coagulation in the heart-lung machine, 500 IU heparin were given in the perfusate. The flow into the liver was 300–600 ml/min. The perfusate was heated to 41 °C and oxygenated. Results of blood gas analysis and levels of blood sugar and electrolytes in the perfusate are shown in Table 4.

Conclusion

Isolated hepatic liver perfusion (IHLP) represents a treatment alternative for irresectable liver tumors. Up to now clinical experience with this method is very limited. The procedure presents a variety of problems to the anesthetist with regard to hemodynamics, coagulation (Bornscheuer et al. 1996), electrolytes, fluid and acid-base balance.

Our first result with IHLP indicate that, under the conditions of elevated monitoring, complete isolation of the liver, a good wash-out and safe anesthe-

Table 4. Liver metabolism during perfusion

	Before therapy	After therapy
Sodium (mmol/l)	147.4	151.8
Potassium (mmol/l)	8.05	5.38
Calcium (mmol/l)	0.45	0.66
Hematocrit (%)	18	14
Hemoglobin (g/dl)	6.1	4.8
Blood sugar (mmol/l)	8.5	25
Saturation (%)	97.8	97.7
pH	6.82	6.926
PCO2 (mmHg)	1.7	5.8
PO2 (mmHg)	292.1	210.1
HCO_3 (mmol/l)	0.3	1.1
Flow (ml/min)		600

siological management, no major disturbances must be expected during the therapy. The patients are more compromised by the therapy during the following days. Low diastolic blood pressure and loss of resistance after perfusion were the first signs of a toxic reaction. Except in the case of one patient with a compromised coagulation status at the beginning of the operation, coagulation conditions after therapy were stable in all patients. All other recorded data were the same after therapy as preoperatively. The high temperature required in IHLP turned out to be less of a problem than in patients with intraperitoneal hyperthermic perfusion (Sudarshan and Crawford 1992).

References

Aigner KR, Walther H, Tonn JC, Link KH, Schoch P, Schwemmle K (1984) Isolated liver perfusion in advanced metastases of colorectal cancer. Onkologie 7:13–21

Arnestad JP, Bengtsson A, Bentson JP, Henriksson BA, Stenqvist O, Naredi P, Hafström L (1992) Isolated hyperthermic liver perfusion with cytostatic-containing perfusate activates the complement cascade. Br J Surg 79:948–951

Bornscheuer A, Mahr KH, Oldhafer KJ, Höltje M, Szabo M, Goldmann R, Lang H, Nadalin S (1996) Coagulation disorders after isolated hyperthermic liver perfusion with Mitomycin C. In: Proceedings, International Hepato Pancreato Biliary Association. I. Liver. Monduzzi, Bologna, pp 367–370

Craft PS, Pembrey RG (1987) Veno-occlusive disease of the liver following chemotherapy with mitomycin C and doxorubicin. Aust N Z J Med 17:449–451

Hafström LR, Holmberg SB, Naredi PL, Lindner PG, Bengtsson A, Tiedebrandt G, Schersten TS (1994) Isolated hyperthermic liver perfusion with chemotherapy for liver malignancy. Surg Oncol 3:103–108

Quebbeman EJ, Skibba JL, Petroff RJ (1984) A technique for isolated hyperthermic liver perfusion. J Surg Oncol 27:141–145

Sudarshan G, Crawford D (1992) Anaesthesia for intraperitoneal hyperthermic perfusion. Anaesthesia 47:483–485

Takayasu K, Makuuchi M, Moriya Y (1990) Portal vein obstruction complicating intraarterial chemo-infusion for hepatic metastases. J Gastroenterol Hepatol 5:708–713

Verweij J, Stoter G (1987) Severe side effects of the cytotoxic drug mitomycin C. Neth J Med 30:43–50

III. High-Dose Chemoperfusion

Percutaneous Isolated Liver Chemoperfusion for Treatment of Unresectable Malignant Liver Tumors: Technique, Pharmacokinetics, Clinical Results

Y. Ku, T. Iwasaki, T. Fukumoto, M. Tominaga, S. Muramatsu,
N. Kusunoki, T. Sugimoto, Y. Suzuki, Y. Kuroda, and Y. Saitoh

First Department of Surgery, Kobe University School of Medicine,
7-5-2 Kusunoki-cho, Chuo-ku, Kobe 650, Japan

Abstract

We have developed a single-catheter technique for percutaneous isolated liver chemoperfusion (PILP) with hepatic venous isolation and charcoal hemoperfusion (HVI-CHP) for the treatment of malignant liver tumors. We report here the surgical technique, pharmacokinetics, and effectiveness of PILP in multiple advanced liver tumors. Twenty-eight patients with hepatocellular carcinoma (HCC) and 18 with metastatic liver tumors underwent a total of 61 PILPs with HVI-CHP. HVI-CHP was accomplished mainly by the single-catheter technique using a novel four-lumen, two-balloon catheter; it was used to isolate and capture total hepatic venous outflow and, at the same time, to direct the filtered blood to the right atrium. Under HVI-CHP, either doxorubicin (60–150 mg/m^2) or cisplatin (150–200 mg/m^2) was infused via the hepatic artery. The PILP was completed successfully in all 61 trials. Two of forty-six patients died early; one of necrotizing pancreatitis and the other of hepatic arterial thrombosis. Both deaths were related directly to the hepatic arterial catheter. Excluding these two deaths, the treatments were well tolerated. The major side effects were mild to moderate chemical hepatitis and reversible myelosuppression. Of the 27 evaluable HCC patients, 17 (63%) had an objective tumor response (5 complete and 12 partial responses). In 15 patients with colorectal hepatic metastases (CHM), 7 had a sharp decrease in serum carcinoembryonic antigen (CEA) levels (to $<50\%$ of their pretreatment levels) after treatment. However, a single PILP had limited efficacy in terms of the durability of remission (≤ 6 months in most CHM patients, as assessed by CEA levels). These results indicate that PILP with HVI-CHP has high efficacy in most patients with multiple advanced liver tumors. In addition, the results suggest a role of multiple treatment courses of PILP in the induction of long-term remission, especially for patients responsive to the first treatment.

Recent Results in Cancer Research, Vol. 147

Introduction

Isolated liver perfusion (ILP) with high-dose chemotherapeutic agents has been attempted for treatment of malignant liver tumors over several decades by a number of investigators (Creech et al. 1958; Aigner 1988).

Despite its potential efficacy, ILP is an extensive procedure and has precluded wide acceptance in clinical use.

As an alternative, we previously developed a less invasive, percutaneous technique of ILP combining hepatic arterial infusion (HAI) chemotherapy with extracorporeal drug elimination by hepatic venous isolation and charcoal hemoperfusion (HVI-CHP). This percutaneous ILP (PILP) allows major dose intensification in HAI chemotherapy with reduced systemic toxicity (Ku et al. 1989, 1990). Our phase I clinical studies have shown that the maximum tolerated dose of doxorubicin was about 150 mg/m^2 and that response rates reached 50–64% with a single treatment in patients with malignant liver tumors (Ku et al. 1995, 1996). After introduction of a unique four-lumen, two-balloon (4L/2B) catheter, the HVI-CHP technique was further simplified (Ku et al. 1997) and PILP could be performed repeatedly in the same patient. Herein we describe the surgical technique, pharmacokinetics, and indications for PILP and report its effectiveness in patients with regionally advanced liver tumors.

Patients and Methods

Indication

Over an 8-year period beginning in May 1989, a group of 46 patients with regionally advanced liver tumors underwent a total of 61 PILPs with HVI-CHP. Altogether 28 patients had hepatocellular carcinoma (HCC), 15 colorectal hepatic metastasis (CHM), and the remaining 3 metastatic breast cancer ($n=2$) and malignant melanoma ($n=1$) (Table 1). All 46 patients had multiple liver tumors deemed unresectable and intractable with currently available therapies.

Regardless of the etiology of liver tumors, patients had to meet the following criteria: no preexisting heart disease, a Karnofsky's performance rating of 40% or more, serum bilirubin level <2.5 mg/dl, 15-min indocyanine green retention rate <35%, serum aspartate aminotransferase (AST) level <300 IU/L, platelet count >50000/mm^3, no episodes of hepatic encephalopathy, and no esophageal varices at risk for bleeding.

HAI Catheter Placement

In the angiography suite the left groin (for the first and second PILPs) or the right groin (for the third and fourth PILPs) is prepared, and the common fe-

Table 1. Indications for PILP with HVI-CHP in 46 patients with unresectable liver tumors

Liver tumor	No. of patients	No. of PILPs
Hepatocellular carcinoma	28	39
Metastatic lesions	18	22
Colorectal	15	19
Breast	2	2
Melanoma	1	1

PILP, percutaneous isolated lever chemoperfusion; *HVI-CHP,* hepatic venous isolation and charcoal hemoperfusion

moral artery is punctured. With use of the Seldinger technique, an HAI catheter is placed in the proper hepatic artery after mapping the vascular supply to the liver by celiac and superior mesenteric arteriography. Whenever possible, the right gastric artery and gastroduodenal arteries are embolized with coils to avoid the risk of drug malperfusion to the stomach, small bowel, and pancreas. The HAI catheter is secured in place, and the patient is immediately transferred to the operating room.

Anesthetic Management

All patients are positioned on a heating blanket set at 38 °C. After induction of general endotracheal anesthesia by thiamylal and vecuronium, the patient is mechanically ventilated with a nitrous oxide/oxygen mixture (60%/40%). Immediately before HVI-CHP, the patient is rapidly given lactated Ringer's solution 10–20 ml/kg along with 1000–1500 ml of 4.4% albumin intravenously. During HVI-CHP dopamine is used at a dose ranging from 5 to 20 μg/kg per minute, and a muscle relaxant is given frequently to prevent depletion due to its binding to the filters. The patient is continuously monitored by electrocardiography as well as central venous pressure and arterial pressure measurements. At the end of the procedure the patient is given diuretics and is then extubated. Intravenous 5% dextrose is given during the first 12 h. Oral intake is allowed the following morning.

PILP with HVI-CHP: Surgical Technique

The femoral vein is exposed 2–3 cm above the saphenofemoral junction through a small cut-down incision on the groin opposite the HAI catheter insertion site. For repeated treatment the femoral vein can be exposed above the inguinal ligament. The patient is then given heparin 100 U/kg IV, and the activated clotting time is maintained above 200 s during the procedure.

A 4L/2B catheter (Fig. 1) is inserted into the femoral vein after a cut-down incision and gently advanced under fluoroscopic guidance until the cephalad balloon is above the diaphragmatic hiatus. During placement an angio-

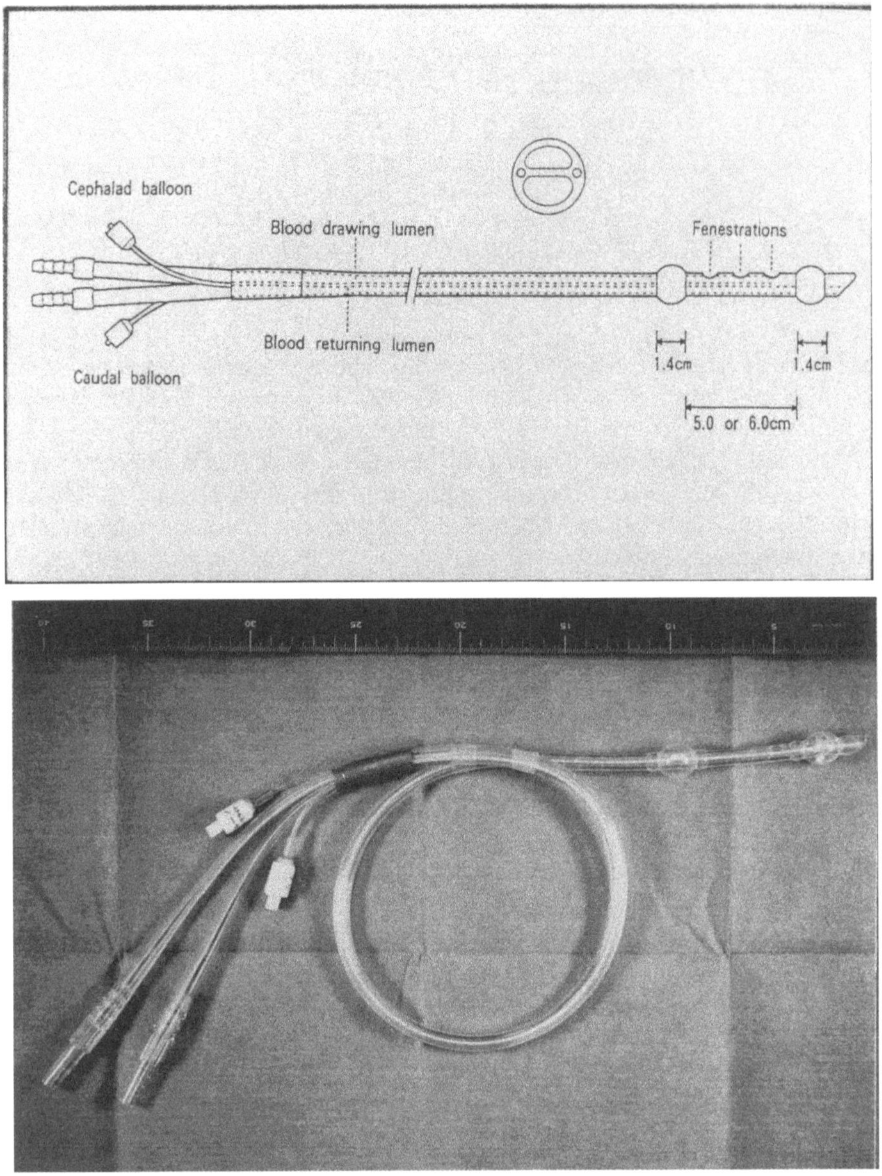

Fig. 1. Four-lumen/two-balloon catheter (24F/26F, respectively). The catheter is 70 cm in length, is radiopaque, and has two occlusion balloons, both of which expand to a maximum of 3 cm diameter. The interballoon segment has three fenestrations in one major lumen. The other major lumen has an opening at the catheter tip. Two accessory lumens are separately used for balloon inflation

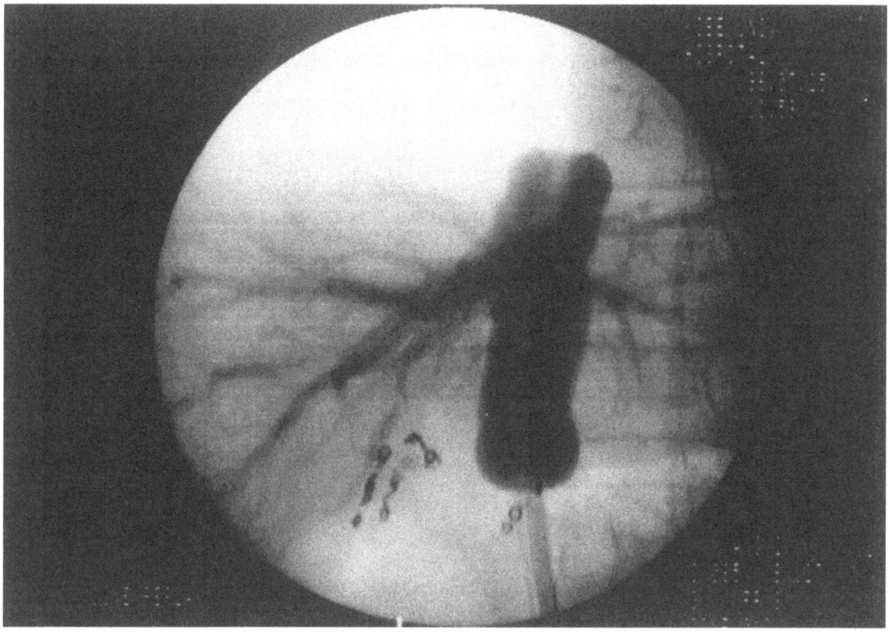

Fig. 2. Venogram obtained during hepatic venous isolation. Contrast agent was injected through one major lumen with fenestra between the balloons

graphic guidewire is used when resistance to the catheter advancement is felt. Under fluoroscopic control, the cephalad balloon is positioned at the suprahepatic inferior vena cava and inflated with 7–12 ml of half-strength contrast agent. To determine the appropriate position of the cephalad balloon, 30 ml of full-strength contrast agent is injected through one major lumen with fenestrations between the balloons. After demonstrating retrograde filling of the hepatic venous system, the occlusion is released. When the cephalad balloon's position is considered appropriate, venography is again performed with the cephalad and caudal balloons (8–14 ml), both inflated, to confirm complete hepatic venous isolation (Fig. 2).

The blood-drawing and returning lumens of the 4L/2B catheter are connected to the inflow and outflow tubing of the extracorporeal pump–CHP unit, respectively (Fig. 3). After initiating blood flow through the bypass circuit, the cephalad and caudal balloons are sequentially inflated to achieve complete HVI. During this test period, the patient's blood pressure and heart rate are carefully monitored. If progressive hypotension below 70 mmHg (systolic blood pressure) is noted or if bradycardia below 50 beats per minute is encountered, both balloons are deflated and further fluid or inotropic agent supports are added.

After ascertaining hemodynamic stability, blood flow is switched from the CHP filter-excluded shunt to the CHP filter-containing unit. After reconfirming selective liver perfusion via the HAI catheter, continuous HAI of a che-

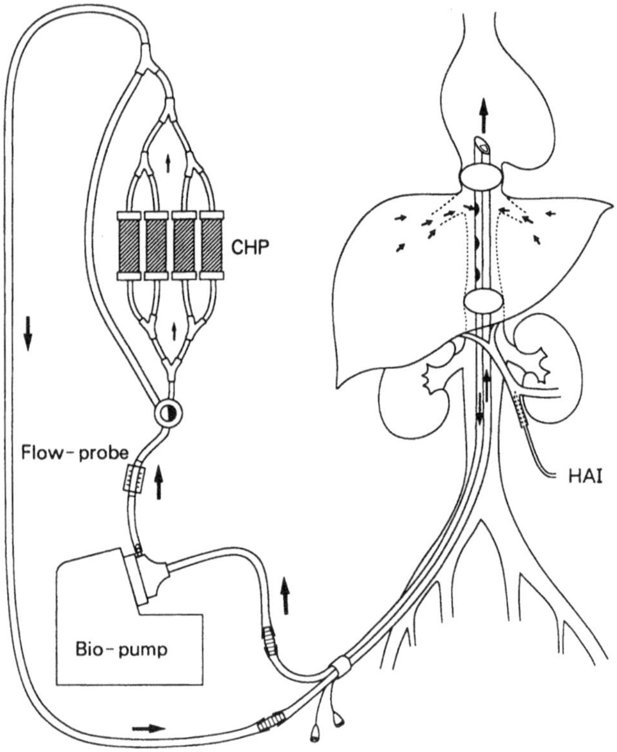

Fig. 3. Bypass circuit of percutaneous isolated liver chemoperfusion (PILP) with hepatic venous isolation and charcoal hemoperfusion (HVI-*CHP).* After hepatic venous isolation, hepatic venous outflow is first directed to the filter-excluded shunt. After ascertaining hemodynamic stability, the blood flow is switched over to the filter-containing route, and hepatic arterial infusion *(HAI)* of a chemotherapeutic agent is initiated

motherapeutic agent (doxorubicin 15–20 min cisplatin 30–40 min) is initiated, and the contour and position of the two balloons are intermittently checked. HVI-CHP is maintained for at least 10 min after the end of HAI. After completion, balloons are deflated, and blood bypass is stopped. The 4L/2B catheter is removed and the femoral vein repaired.

Drugs and Doses

The chemotherapeutic agents and doses are shown in Table 2. Doxorubicin was initially chosen as a first-line agent irrespective of the etiology of the disease. However, in the six most recent PILP trials cisplatin was used at doses of 150 or 200 mg/m^2.

The first dose of doxorubicin ranged from 60 to 150 mg/m^2, (mean 110 mg/m^2). For the second to fourth treatments the dose was reduced to 90 mg/m^2 if the pretreatment leukocyte count was 3000–4000/mm^3 and to 60 mg/m^2

Table 2. Drugs and doses

Drug and dose (mg/m ^{2})	No. of PILPs
Doxorubicin	
60–90	11
100–130	43
150	1
Cisplatin	
150	3
200	3

if the count was 2500–3000/mm ^{3}. In patients with a count below 2500/mm ^{3}, treatment was withdrawn. Repeat treatment was scheduled at 3- to 5-week intervals.

Pharmacokinetic Study

During PILP with HVI-CHP, blood samples were obtained from the filter inlet and outlet and the radial artery (systemic level) at 5- to 10-min intervals. After centrifugation (1000 *g* for 10 min at 4 °C), the plasma was removed and kept on ice. Doxorubicin concentrations in plasma were determined by high-performance liquid chromatography (HPLC) as described previously (Robert 1980). For the cisplatin assay 1 ml plasma was transferred to an ultrafiltration YMT membrane system (Centrifree MPS-3; Amicon, Beverly, MA, USA) and centrifuged at 1000*g* at 4 °C for 20 min. The ultrafiltrates and plasma samples were analyzed directly by flameless absorption spectroscopy to determine the free and total platinum concentrations, as described elsewhere (LeRoy et al. 1977).

Evaluation of Tumor Response and Data Analysis

Postoperative examinations and follow-up studies were performed according to a protocol established previously (Ku et al. 1995). The tumor responses were evaluated by comparison of pretreatment computed tomographic (CT) findings and serum α-fetoprotein (AFP) or carcinoembryonic antigen (CEA) levels with those obtained 1 month after treatment and at 1- to 3-month intervals thereafter. Standard response criteria were used to measure the response (complete remission when all liver tumors disappeared, partial response when the tumor volume was reduced by $>50\%$, stable disease when there was no change, and progressive disease when there was an increase in tumor size). Survival was measured from the date of the first PILP to the time of death or the latest follow-up visit. Response duration (complete and partial) was measured from the date of response recognition to the time of progression of the disease, death, or the date the patient was last known to be in remission. Survival and response duration were calculated by the Kaplan-Meier method.

Results

Hemodynamic Data

Most patients had a smooth, stepwise induction of PILP with HVI-CHP. However, during the first treatment of the HVI test period 5 of 46 patients developed progressive hypotension that required deflating the balloons. In these patients the test for HVI was repeated with additional fluid or inotropic agent support. The hemodynamic profile for one of these five patients is shown in Fig. 4. Once HAI of chemotherapeutic agent was initiated, all 46 patients showed hemodynamic stability, and PILP with HVI-CHP was successfully completed in all 61 trials. There were no procedure-related fatal complications in our series.

The hepatic venous flow rates were remarkably stable, averaging 570±115 ml/min mean±SD during HVI-CHP with use of a 4L/2B catheter. Most patients showed significant decreases in central venous pressure (about 40% of

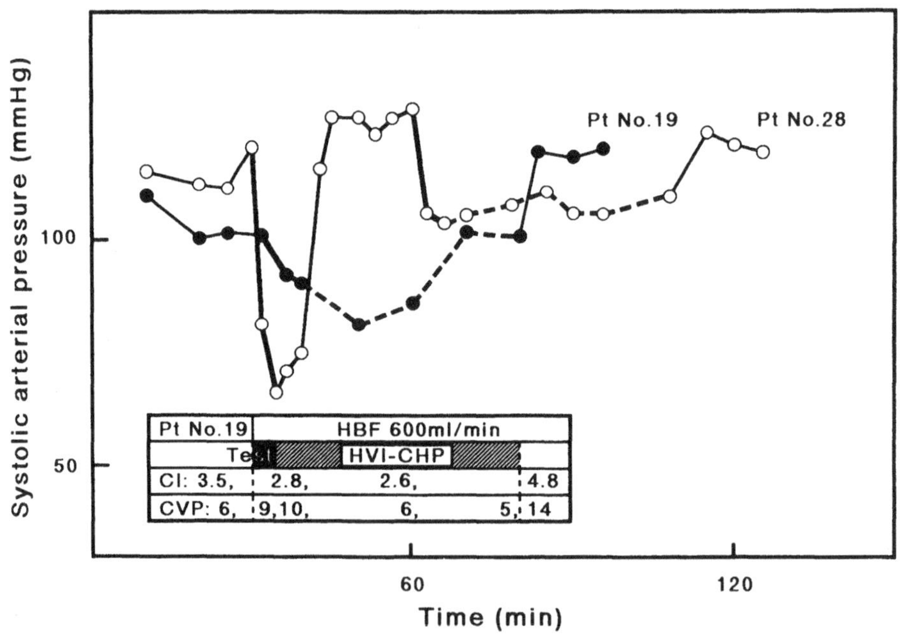

Fig. 4. Hemodynamic changes before, during, and after PILP. *Closed circles* represent a smooth stepwise induction of PILP in patient 19, *open circles* show a hemodynamic profile in patient 28, requiring repeated preconditioning for HVI-CHP. *Dotted lines* indicate the period of HVI-CHP. *HBF,* hepatic blood flow; *CI,* cardiac index; *CVP,* central venous pressure

baseline level) and cardiac output (about 65% of baseline level) during HVI-CHP.

Pharmacokinetic Data

During drug infusion, the CHP filter extraction ratio

$$ER = \frac{C_{in} - C_{out}}{C_{in}} \times 100$$

(where C_{in} = drug concentration at the inlet, C_{out} = drug concentration at the outlet) of doxorubicin ranged from 85% to 95%. In general, the ER gradually decreased to 50–60% 10 min after the end of HAI. The amount of drug removed by HVI-CHP

$$\text{Drug clearance fraction} = \frac{\sum (C_{in} - C_{out}) \times Q \times \Delta T}{\text{amount of drug administered}}$$

(where Q = the hepatic venous flow rate) ranged from 6.5% to 72.3% of the amount of drug administered. Fig. 5A shows a plasma profile of doxorubicin in a patient receiving doxorubicin 100 mg/m^2.

In contrast, the ER of platinum was in a range of 50–94%. The drug clearance fraction ranged from 30% to 59% for total platinum. The Plasma profile of total platinum in one patient administered cisplatin 200 mg/m^2 is shown in Fig. 5B.

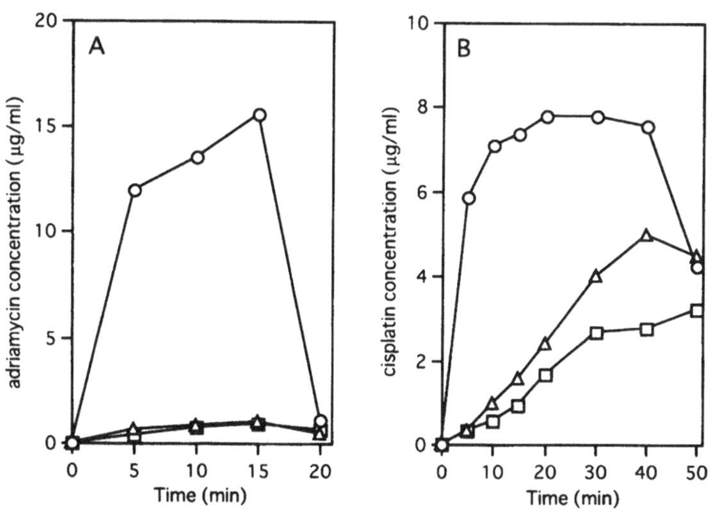

Fig. 5 A, B. Time–concentration curves. (**A**) Serum levels of doxorubicin in a patient with a 15-min HAI of doxorubicin 100 mg/m^2. (**B**) Serum levels of cisplatin in a patient with a 40-min HAI of cisplatin 200 mg/m^2. -○- prefilter; -□- postfilter; -△- systemic

Table 3. Tumor response in 28 patients with hepatocellular carcinoma

Response	No. of patients	
Complete	5/27 (19%)	63%
Partial	12/27 (44%)	
Stable disease	7/27 (26%)	
Progressive disease	3/27 (11%)	
Not evaluable	1	

Tumor Response and Survival

The tumor responses of HCC patients are outlined in Table 3. Data on the one patient who died of necrotizing pancreatitis 1 month after treatment were excluded from the response assessment. The overall (complete and partial) response rate was 63% (17/27 evaluable patients). Figure 6 shows CT findings before and 10 months after repeated PILP in one male patient with a partial response. Five patients had complete remission. Except for one who died at 8 months owing to pulmonary metastases, four patients with complete remission are well and disease-free at 21, 25, 28, and 43 months, respectively, after the first treatment. The 1- and 5-year survivals were 68% and 40%, respectively.

Among 18 patients with metastatic liver tumors, one with breast cancer and one with malignant melanoma had a partial response. However, the mode of response of colorectal hepatic metastasis to PILP was different from those observed in patients with HCC or other metastatic disease. In 9 of 15 patients with colorectal metastases, liver tumors developed liquefaction after treatment, as represented in Fig. 7. Among these nine patients, seven showed a rapid decline in serum CEA values to below 50% of the pretreatment value by 2 months. Although the CEA levels tended to rise again within 3 months in most patients with a single PILP, two patients with repeated PILP with cisplatin showed low CEA levels for 6 months after treatment (Fig. 8).

Complications and Toxicities

Fatal complications relating to the HAI catheter occurred in two early patients with HCC. Except for these two patients, no deaths could be directly or indirectly ascribed to PILP, and the treatment was well tolerated irrespective of the etiology of the liver tumors.

Table 4 lists doxorubicin toxicities. The most freuquent side effect was chemical hepatitis, as indicated by serum aspartate aminotransferase (AST) elevations ranging from 2 to 26 times the baseline level. AST generally reached a peak within 2 days after treatment and decreased promptly to the baseline level after another 2–6 days. All patients had some degree of leuko-

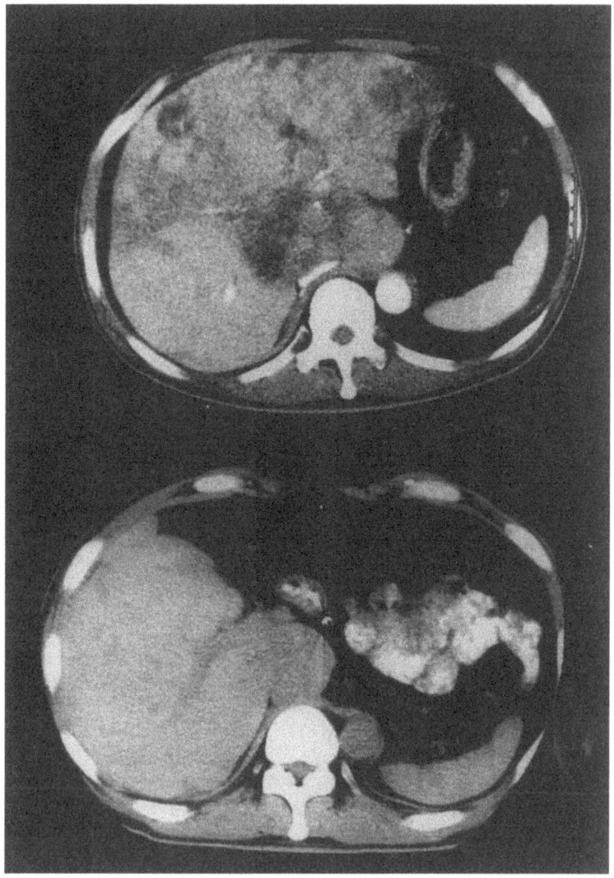

Fig. 6. Computed tomography (CT) findings 1 month *(top)* and 10 months *(bottom)* after the first PILP in a patient with HCC. The patient had a total of two treatments

penias and leukocyte counts below 2000/mm^3 were seen after 24 of 55 trials of PILP with doxorubicin. Nausea and vomiting were encountered after five PILPs. Leukopenia and hair loss were generally more prominent and frequent after repeated PILP. No evidence of cardiac toxicity or sclerosing cholangitis was observed in any patient.

Discussion

The PILP with HVI-CHP technique requires strict attention to the HAI catheter so drug perfusion is applied only to the liver. In one early patient, gastroduodenal misperfusion of doxorubicin occurred. The patient developed frequent nausea and vomiting shortly after treatment, with marked elevation of the serum amylase level. This experience led us to embolize the gastroduode-

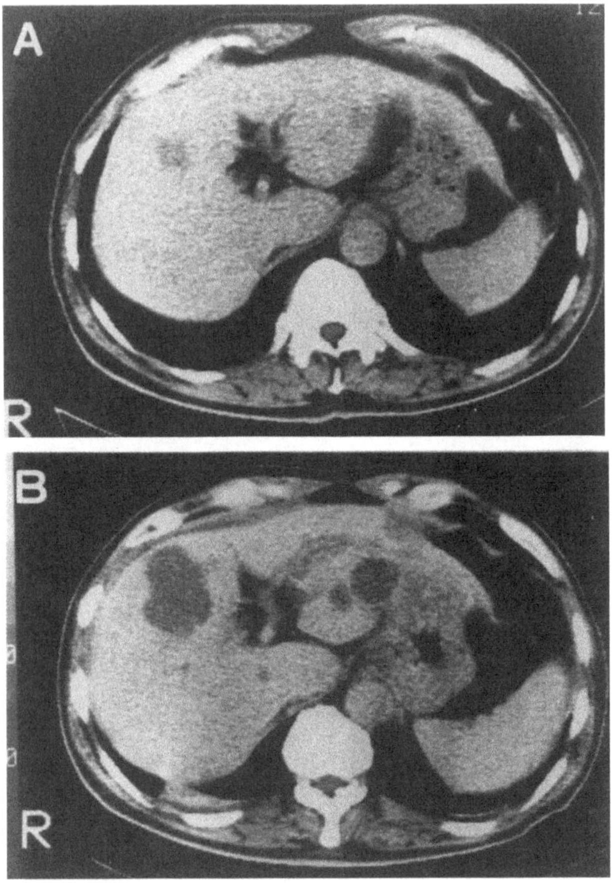

Fig. 7. CT findings before (**A**) and 2 months after (**B**) treatment in a patient with colorectal hepatic metastases. Marked liquefaction of liver tumors was seen after treatment

nal and right gastric arteries with coils, whenever possible, before fixing the tip of the HAI catheter. When we used the right hepatic artery arising from the superior mesenteric artery, the HAI catheter was sufficiently advanced to prevent bowel misperfusion. We also performed a test infusion of contrast agent via the HAI catheter in the middle of drug perfusion to avoid the risk of extrahepatic drug perfusion in such cases.

Other patients experienced hepatic arterial thrombosis 2 months after PILP that was associated with infection caused by the HAI catheter system implanted in the groin. Except for these two fatal complications relating to the HAI catheter, no death was directly or indirectly ascribed to PILP. Another important prerequisite for the success of PILP is careful anesthetic management during the procedure.

Curley et al. (1994) reported a procedure-related death due to acute heart failure in a series of 11 patients, and suggested CHP filter-related cathechola-

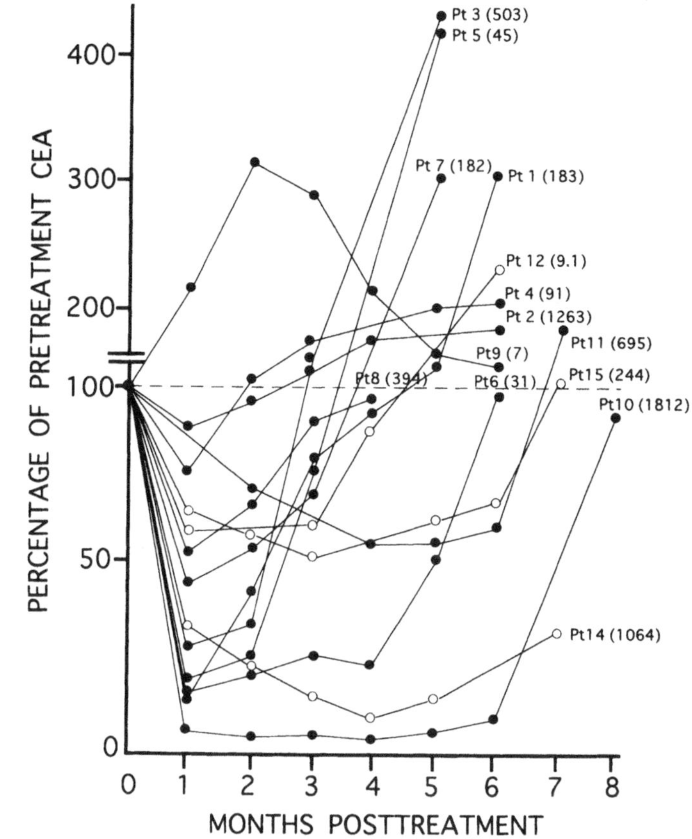

Fig. 8. Percent changes of CEA levels compared with pretreatment levels. -●- single PILP; -○- repeated PILP

mine depletion as a possible cause of the death. Such failure did not occur during the 61 treatments in our series with careful fluid and vasopressor support during HVI-CHP. Apart from the filter-related hypotension, Beheshti et al. (1992) reported severe hypotension during HVI-CHP using the Bodden-Glickman dual-balloon catheter. They speculated that decreased hepatic venous flow due to compression of the catheter lumen by tumor might be the cause of the profound hypotension. In accordance with their experience, significant hypotension was also observed in some patients with a hepatic venous flow rate below 400 ml/min during the HVI-CHP test period. It is important to ensure a stable hepatic venous flow rate, at least above 400 ml/min, before initiating HAI infusion of the drug.

We used doxorubicin as a first-line agent in this series. As illustrated by us (1995) and others (Curley et al. 1993; August et al. 1994), HVI-CHP theoretically offers a greater pharmacologic advantage for a drug such as doxorubicin with a low hepatic extraction ratio. When given by HAI, the system exerts a pharmacologic first-pass effect on a superfluous drug that is not ex-

Table 4. Toxicity associated with 55 PILPs with doxorubicin

Side effect	No. of PILPs
Hematologic: leukocyte count < 2000/mm^3	24 (44%)
Gastrointestinal	
Chemical hepatitis	41 (75%)
Nausea/vomiting	5 (9%)
Ulcer/gastritis	3 (5%)
Sclerosing cholangitis	0
Hair loss	17 (31%)
Cardiac toxicity	0

tracted by the liver. With the aid of the system, we were able to increase the dose of doxorubicin to an average of 110 mg/m^2. Considering significant hepatic and hematologic toxicities, further dose intensification may carry a risk of irreversible myelosuppression. Similar to our findings, Curley et al. (1993) reported the hepatic and systemic maximum tolerated dose to be 120 mg/m^2 based on a phase I study in patients with HCC.

Our previous experimental studies (Maekawa et al. 1993) have shown that HVI-CHP is also applicable to cisplatin. In these experiments the rate of hepatic extraction for cisplatin was lower than that of doxorubicin. As a result, the drug clearance efficiency of HVI-CHP was shown to be greater for cisplatin then for doxorubicin. The pharmacologic data of this study confirmed that cisplatin is a suitable agent for PILP with HVI-CHP in the clinical setting. However, further studies are required to determine the hepatic and systemic maximum tolerated dose of this agent for the system.

Among the HCC patients treated with PILP, 27 were evaluable for tumor response; and 17 had at least a 50% reduction in tumor volume. It is noted that four of five patients with complete remission are still free of disease with completely normalized AFP or PIVKA-II (protein induced by vitamin K absence or antagonism) levels (or both) 21–43 months after treatment. Regardless of therapy, such long-lasting remissions have rarely been reported in patients with extensive tumor burdens. In this study, overall survival rates were 68% at 1 year and 40% at 5 years; the median survival of all 28 patients was 16 months. Among our historical controls with multiple bilobar HCC, the median duration of survival was approximately 6 months, and there were no 5-year survivors. In accordance with our historical data, other investigators reported that the median survival ranged from 3.5 to 6.0 months for patients with unresectable HCCs selected for chemotherapy (Doci et al. 1988; O'Connell et al. 1989). We believe that PILP with HVI-CHP has a significant impact on prolonging survival duration in patients for whom no effective therapy otherwise exists.

In contrast, in 15 patients with multiple CHM, a single PILP with doxorubicin had limited efficacy in terms of the durability of remission, as assessed by serum CEA levels (Ku et al. 1996). In this study, 7 of the 15 patients showed a sharp fall in CEA levels (to <50% of their pretreatment values), but the value tended to rise again in most patients with a single PILP. In contrast, the two most recent patients treated with repeated PILP with high-dose cisplatin have shown low CEA levels during 6 months following the first PILP. Although our experience with repeated PILP using cisplatin is limited, we believe that this regimen holds considerable promise as an inductive treatment for patients with unresectable CHM and for patients with other tumors metastatic to the liver.

References

Aigner KR (1988) Isolated liver perfusion: 5 year results. Reg Cancer Treat 1:11-20

August DA, Verma N, Andrews JC, Vaerten MA, Brenner DE (1994) Hepatic artery infusion of doxorubicin with hepatic venous drug extraction. J Surg Res 56:611-619

Beheshti MV, Denny DF, Glickman MG, Bodden W, Marsh JC, Strair R, Ravikumar TS (1992) Percutaneous isolated liver perfusion for treatment of hepatic malignancy: preliminary report. J Vasc Interv Radiol 3:453-458

Creech O Jr, Kremenz ET, Ryan RF, Winblad JN (1958) Chemotherapy of cancer: regional perfusion utilizing an extracorporeal circuit. Ann Surg 148:616-632

Curley SA, Byrd DR, Newman RA, Ellis HJ, Chase J, Garrasco CH, Cleary K, Bodden W, Hohn DC (1993) Reduction of systemic drug exposure after hepatic arterial infusion of doxorubicin with complete hepatic venous isolation and extracorporeal chemofiltration. Surgery 114:579-585

Curley SA, Newman RA, Dougherty TB, Fuhrman GM, Stone DL, Mikolajek JA, Guercio S, Guercio A, Garrasco CH, Kuo T, Hohn DC (1994) Complete hepatic venous isolation and extracorporeal chemofiltration as treatment for human hepatocellular carcinoma: a phase 1 study. Ann Surg Oncol 1:389-399

Doci R, Bignemi P, Bozzetti F (1988) Intrahepatic chemotherapy for unresectable hepatocellular carcinoma. Cancer 61:1983-1987

Ku Y, Saitoh M, Nishiyama H, Fujiwara S, Iwasaki T, Ohyanagi H, Saitoh Y (1989) Extracorporeal adriamycin removal following hepatic artery infusion: use of direct hemoperfusion combined with veno-venous bypass. J Jpn Surg Soc 90:1758-1764

Ku Y, Saitoh M, Nishiyama H, Fujiwara S, Iwasaki T, Tominaga M, Maekawa Y, Ohyanagi H, Saitoh Y (1990) Extracorporeal removal of anticancer drugs in hepatic artery infusion; the effect of direct hemoperfusion combined with venovenous bypass. Surgery 107:273-281

Ku Y, Fukumoto T, Iwasaki T, Tominaga M, Samizo M, Nishida T, Kuroda Y, Hirota S, Sako M, Obara H, Saitoh Y (1995) Clinical pilot study on high-dose intraarterial chemotherapy with direct hemoperfusion in patients with advanced hepatocellular carcinoma. Surgery 117:510-519

Ku Y, Tominaga M, Iwasaki T, Kitagawa T, Maeda I, Shiotani M, Kusunoki N, Maekawa Y, Samizo M, Fukumoto T, Kuroda Y, Hirota S, Saitoh Y (1996) Percutaneous hepatic venous isolation and extracorporeal charcoal hemoperfusion for high-dose intraarterial chemotherapy in patients with colorectal hepatic metasatases. Surg Today 26:305-313

Ku Y, Fukumoto T, Tominaga M, Iwasaki T, Maeda I, Kusunoki N, Obara H, Sako M, Suzuki Y, Kuroda Y, Saitoh Y (1997) Single catheter technique of hepatic venous isolation and extracorporeal charcoal hemoperfusion for malignant liver tumors. Am J Surg 173:103-109

LeRoy AF, Wehling ML, Sponseller HL, Friauf WS, Solomon RE, Dedrick RL (1977) Analysis of platinum in biological materials by flameless atomic absorption spectrophotometry. Biochem Med 18:184-189

Maekawa Y, Ku Y, Saitoh Y (1993) Extracorporeal cisplatin removal using direct hemoperfusion under hepatic venous isolation for hepatic arterial chemotherapy: an experimental study on pharmacokinetics. Surg Today 23:58–62

O'Connell MJ, Hahn RG, Rubin J (1989) Chemotherapy of malignant hepatomas with sequential intraarterial doxorubicin and systemic 5-fluorouracil and semustine. Cancer 62:1041–1043

Robert J (1980) Extraction of anthracyclines from biologic fluids for HPLC evaluation. J Liquid Chromatogr 3:1561–1572

Phase I/II Studies of Isolated Hepatic Perfusion with Mitomycin C or Melphalan in Patients with Colorectal Cancer Hepatic Metastases

A. Marinelli, A.L. Vahrmeijer, and C.J.H. van de Velde

Department of Surgery, Leiden University Medical Center, Postal Zone K6-R, PO Box 9600, 2300 RC, Leiden, The Netherlands

Abstract

In an attempt to improve tumor response and survival among patients with colorectal cancer metastases confined to the liver, we developed an experimental (rats and pigs) and clinical isolated hepatic perfusion (IHP) technique to exploit maximally the steep dose-response relation of many anticancer drugs. In this overview we present our experimental and clinical results with mitomycin C (MMC) and melphalan (L-PAM). In rats, treatment with a four times higher maximally tolerated dose (MTD) of MMC during IHP compared to hepatic artery infusion (HAI) resulted in higher, more effective intratumoral concentrations of MMC. As a result, only in the IHP-treated rats were complete remissions observed and long-term survival achieved. Hepatotoxic side effects were minimal and transient in all animals. In the clinical phase I/II study with MMC 30 mg/m^2 administrated as a bolus in the isolated circuit, two of nine patients had a complete remission, with a median survival of 17 months. Four patients developed venoocclusive disease (VOD) of the liver, and as a result one patient died. Therefore we consider MMC unsuitable for further IHP studies. Meanwhile experiments in rats showed that IHP with the L-PAM MTD of 12 mg/kg was even more effective than MMC and did not cause hepatotoxic side effects. In the phase I/II dose-finding study with L-PAM in IHP, the MTD in humans was approximately 3.0 mg/kg. As in the rats, systemic toxicity was dose-limiting. The median survival of the whole group was 18 months. We have started a phase II study of L-PAM in IHP with a fixed dose of 200 mg L-PAM to determine if IHP can significantly increase the median survival and complete remission rate compared to other treatment modalities. Results from this study are expected by the end of 1997.

Introduction

Hepatic metastases are a major cause of death of colorectal cancer patients. The liver is a primary site of dissemination, and liver involvement largely determines prognosis (Wanebo et al. 1978). Knowledge about colorectal cancer

Recent Results in Cancer Research, Vol. 147

has much increased, but little progress has been made in improvement of patient survival, especially for patients with liver metastases. Up to now surgery has been the only hope for prolonged survival. The selection criteria for surgery of colorectal hepatic metastases are (I) no primary colorectal tumor left, (2) metastases confined to the liver, and (3) resection possible with tumor-free margins of all metastases. Thus only 5–10% of all colorectal cancer patients are candidates for resection. A 5-year survival rate of 25–35% can be obtained after radical resection of hepatic metastases (van Ooijen et al. 1992; Vahrmeijer et al. 1995). With no therapy the 5-year survival of these patients is negligible. Systemic chemotherapy results in objective tumor responses in approximately 25% of patients with liver metastases but does not improve survival significantly (Kemeny 1995; Vahrmeijer et al. 1995; Sobrero et al. 1997).

Attempting to improve the response rate and survival of patients with unresectable colorectal cancer metastases confined to the liver, many trials aimed at increasing drug exposure at the target side. Various drug targeting modalities have been developed that expose liver metastases more selectively to higher drug concentrations, thereby exploiting the steep dose–response relation of most anticancer drugs, while systemic toxicity remains tolerable. Because hepatic metastases derive most of their blood supply from the hepatic artery (Ackerman et al. 1969; Wang et al. 1994), hepatic artery infusion is used extensively as a method of treatment. Indeed, this treatment produced a significant increase in response rates of hepatic metastases from colorectal carcinoma when compared with systemic treatment in six randomized studies (Meta-Analysis Group in Cancer 1996). In a more recent study hepatic artery infusion resulted in a significantly longer median survival rate (Kemeny et al. 1994). To be able to treat liver metastases with still higher doses of anticancer drugs, various isolated liver perfusion techniques have been developed in pigs, rats, and humans (van de Velde et al. 1986; Aigner et al. 1988; de Brauw et al. 1991; Marinelli et al. 1991 a–c, 1996; Hafstrom et al. 1994). With this technique the liver is completely isolated vascularly so as to recirculate anticancer agents only through the liver and liver metastases. The advantage of this approach is that systemic toxicity is not a factor that limits the use of high drug dosages.

We studied three drugs: 5-fluorouracil (5FU), mitomycin C (MMC), and melphalan (L-PAM). 5-FU was used because it is still considered the standard drug for the treatment of advanced colorectal cancer (Sobrero et al. 1997); MMC because its response rate is comparable to that with 5-FU and has been used with some success as a salvage treatment for patients with hepatic metastases of colorectal cancer (Doll et al. 1985); and L-PAM because of its associated surprisingly high overall response rate in patients with colon cancer after high-dose L-PAM plus autologous bone marrow transplantation (Lazarus et al. 1983). In this overview we present data from our rat and human studies with MMC and L-PAM.

Isolated Hepatic Perfusion Technique in Rats

The tumor model used in the rat experiments is based on the CC531 colorectal adenocarcinoma. The syngeneic CC531 tumor cell line was established from a colorectal adenocarcinoma induced by dimethylhydrazine in a male Wistar rat (Marquet et al. 1984). When injected subcapsularly in the liver these cells rapidly grow out into solid tumors. With the isolated hepatic perfusion technique in rats, the inflow limbs consist of the cannulated pyloric vein and gastroduodenal artery. The outflow consists of a cannula in the intrahepatic caval vein, which is temporarily ligated just above and below the liver. To complete isolation, the infradiaphragmatic aorta, distal portal vein, and common hepatic artery are clamped. During the 25 min of isolated perfusion the intestines are cooled with melting ice.

The perfusion circuit (Fig. 1) consisted of two low-flow roller pumps (Watson Marlow; de Jong B.V., Rotterdam, The Netherlands), a specially constructed heat exchanger, and an oxygenator, all fitted with PVC tubing. The recirculating system was primed with 30 ml Haemaccel (Hoechst, Amsterdam, The Netherlands) and added heparin (50 U), and the pH was kept be-

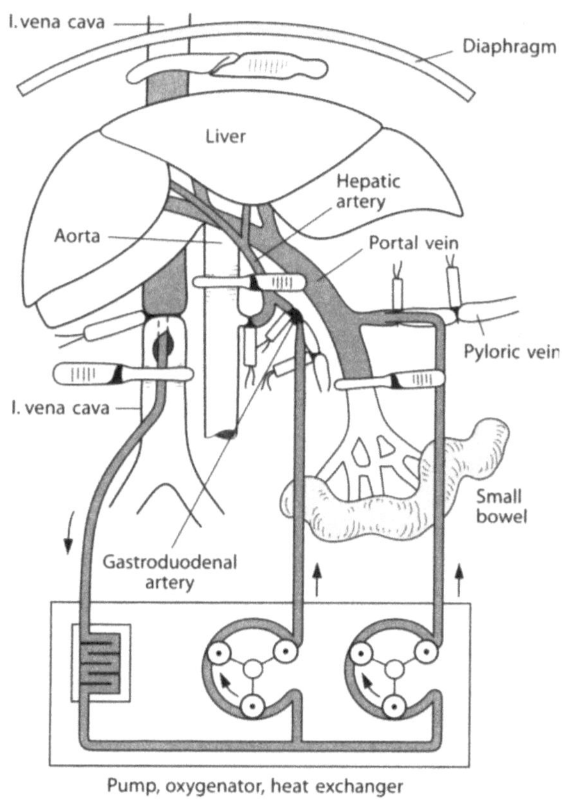

Fig. 1. Isolated hepatic perfusion circuit in the rat

tween 7.3 and 7.4 using bicarbonate (0.5–1.0 ml 8.4% potassium bicarbonate). The perfusate was infused into the pyloric branch of the portal vein at a flow rate of 20 ml/min and in the gastroduodenal branch of the common hepatic artery at a flow rate of 4.5 ml/min. The hepatic venous outflow was collected by an intracaval cannula and was returned to the oxygenator by gravity feed. The perfusate was gassed during perfusion with a mixture of (O_2/CO_2 (95%/5%) at a flow rate of 50 ml/min. The perfusate temperature was kept at 38 °±0.5 °C. At the end of the procedure a washout was performed with 8 ml saline (37 °C), which was perfused through the liver using the pyloric vein cannula only. Total operating time was 2.0–2.5 h.

Isolated Heptic Perfusion Technique in Humans

Original Technique

To control the suprahepatic caval vein the liver is mobilized from the diaphragm, identifiable diaphragm veins are ligated, the pericardium is opened by incising the diaphragm just anterior to the caval vein, and the caval vein is dissected free of adhering tissue and secured with tape. Lumbar veins are identified and transected. The common bile duct, portal vein, common hepatic artery, and gastroduodenal artery are dissected from the hepatoduodenal ligament. The common bile duct, common hepatic artery, and gastric artery branches are clamped during perfusion. The infrahepatic caval vein is dissected free of adhering tissue proximal and distal to the renal veins. After heparinization, the intrahepatic caval vein is cannulated with a specially designed double-lumen catheter (Braun, Melsungen, Germany), which is inserted/introduced just distal to the renal veins. The longer, central lumen allows undisturbed blood flow from the infrahepatic caval vein to the heart and has side ports for a temporary portocaval shunt and for the renal veins. The outer, shorter lumen collects the hepatic venous outflow. The portal vein and gastroduodenal artery (and if present an aberrant hepatic artery) are cannulated to establish the venous and arterial inflow limbs of the isolated circuit (Fig. 2).

After establishing vascular isolation, perfusion is started. The hepatic venous outflow (perfusate consists of intrahepatically trapped blood and 1 l Haemaccel) is collected and returned to an oxygenator, a reservoir, and a heat excanger (37 °±1 °C). Two roller pumps infuse the perfusate into the liver via the portal vein (flow 320 ml/min) and the hepatic artery (flow 400 ml/min). Leakage from and to the extracorporeal circuit is monitored by adding radio-labeled technetium(^{99m}Tc) red blood cells to the perfusate and placing detectors in the extracorporeal circuit and the systemic circulation (Runia et al. 1987) MMC and L-PAM are added after leakage has been excluded. After 1 h of perfusion with the cytostatics, washout is performed using 3 l of Haemaccel, the shunt is removed, and normal circulation is reestablished.

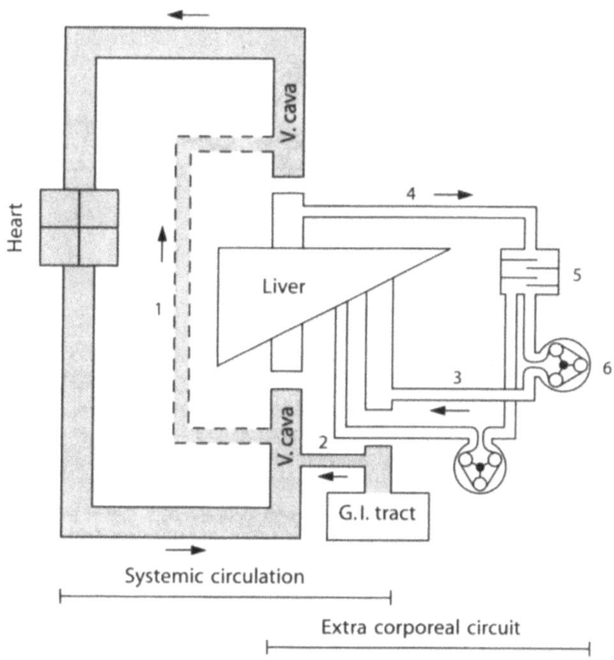

Fig. 2. Perfusion circuit: *(1)* intracaval double-lumen shunt, *(2)* portacaval shunt; *(3)* inflow limbs of the perfusion circuit infusing into the common hepatic artery and the portal vein; *(4)* hepatic venous outflow returning the perfusate to *(5)* reservoir + heat exchanger and *(6)* two roller pumps

Changed Technique

With the altered technique, the before-mentioned double-lumen catheter placed in the intrahepatic caval vein is replaced by a single outflow cannula in the intrahepatic caval vein, and the caval vein is clamped suprahepatically (infradiaphragmally) and infrahepatically. Furthermore, the blood of the lower body-half is shunted by a biomed pump from the portal vein and left common iliac vein to the left axillary vein (Fig. 3).

Isolated Hepatic Perfusion Studies with MMC in Rats and Humans

In our rat tumor model we first demonstrated in a toxicity study that isolated hepatic perfusion (IHP) allowed administration of a four times higher dose of MMC than did hepatic artery infusion (4.8 versus 1.2 mg/kg) and that hepatic, not systemic, toxicity was dose-limiting (Marinelli et al. 1991b). Subsequently we measured MMC concentrations in tumor tissue and showed that in rats treated with the maximally tolerated dose during IHP a significantly (almost fivefold) higher concentration was reached. Interested in the effectiveness of MMC on the growth of individual tumor cells and the whole

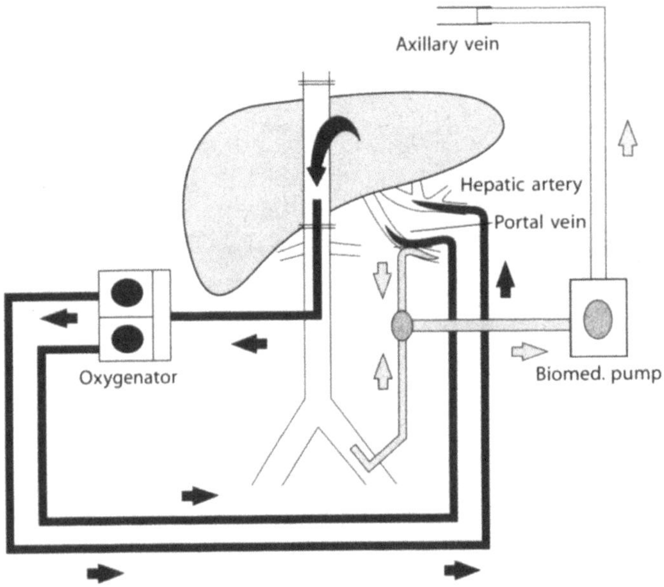

Fig. 3. Isolated hepatic perfusion circuit with extracorporeal venovenous bypass

tumor, we studied cell cycle progression by flow cytometric analysis of cellular DNA contents of tumor cells and in vivo tumor growth (Marinelli et al. 1991a).

It is well known that an increase in intracellular MMC concentration results in a higher number of crosslinks between DNA strands, and that this damage to the DNA inhibits normal DNA replication and may lead to cell death (Crooke and Bradner 1976; Dorr et al. 1985). Flow cytometric analysis of cellular DNA contents of tumor cells 24 h after MMC 4.8 mg/kg via IHP revealed a significant increase in the fraction of tumor cells in the mid and late S-phase, whereas after MMC 1.2 mg/kg via hepatic artery infusion there was no DNA synthesis inhibition. Figure 4 shows the growth patterns of CC531 tumors. Tumor growth was not influenced by perfusion without MMC. In most rats the tumors had reached a lethal size at day 42. After treatment with the maximally tolerated dose of MMC in IHP five of seven rats showed complete remission from day 14 until sacrifice. In one rat one tumor regressed but relapsed between days 14 and 28, whereas the other tumor showed a minimal growth delay during the first 14 days. No growth inhibition was observed in the second nonresponding rat. Based on these preclinical data and on the study reported by Aigner et al. (1988), a phase I/II study was started with MMC 30 mg/m^2 in the IHP setting (Marinelli et al. 1996). This study was approved by the Medical Ethics Committee of the Leiden Medical Center. From May 1990 to May 1991 nine patients with unresectable hepatic metastases of colon cancer scattered throughout the liver were selected. The preoperative workup consisted of a control coloscopy, com-

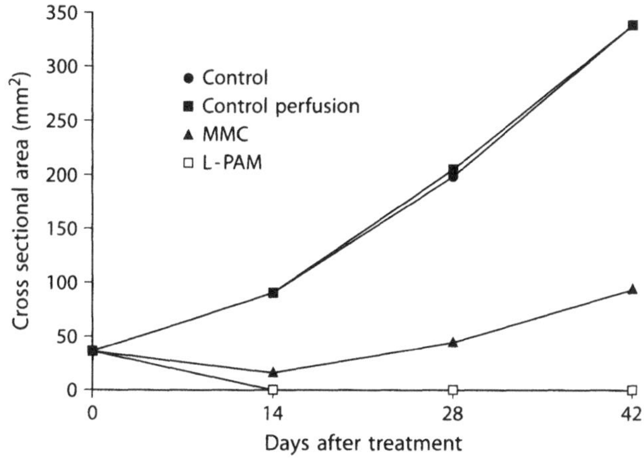

Fig. 4. Growth curves of CC531 liver tumors after melphalan (L-PAM) or mitomycin C (*MMC*) treatment at the maximally tolerated dose administrated via isolated hepatic perfusion

puted tomographic (CT) scan of the abdomen, a chest radiograph, and routine laboratory tests plus carcinoembryonic antigen (CEA) level. With informed consent, all patients underwent IHP at the Leiden University Medical Center.

Complete remission was seen in two of nine patients as measured from the CT scan in one and at autopsy in the other (the only patient who died from venoocclusive disease). In all patients the 3-month postoperative CEA levels were less than 50% of the preoperative values. Unfortunately, these CEA responses were of short duration (<9 months). The median survival of the nine treated patients was 17 months. As in the rat studies, all patients had a transient increase in plasma levels of liver enzymes and bilirubin. Four patients developed venoocclusive disease (VOD) of the liver. In one patient the VOD was subclinical, in two the symptoms were reversible, and in one the VOD was lethal. Clinical signs of VOD are jaundice, hepatomegaly or right upper quadrant pain (or both), and ascites or unexplained weight gain. Histologically, fibrin immediately surrounds veins and apparently obstructs inflow of blood from sinusoids during early VOD. Loose connective tissue occupies part or all of the lumen, and depending on the extent of venous occlusion it has a subclinical, clinically evident, or even lethal effect. Reports on VOD have rapidly increased since the introduction of high-dose chemotherapy combined with cryopreserved autologous bone marrow transplantation. VOD is probably the most common disease associated with dose-escalation chemotherapy plus bone marrow transplantation, manifesting within 8–20 days (Shulman et al. 1980). VOD has been observed after treatment with high-dose 1,3-bis(2-chloroethyl) 1-nitrosourea (BCNU), arabinosyl cytosine, dimethylbusulfan, and MMC (Gottfried and Sudilovsky 1982; Lazarus et al. 1982). We stopped the IHP study with MMC because of these toxic side effects.

Isolated Hepatic Perfusion with L-PAM in Rats and Humans

In a toxicity study with L-PAM in rats the maximally tolerated dose in the IHP was 12 mg/kg, which is twice as high as that in the hepatic artery infusion (Marinelli et al. 1991c). The L-PAM concentration in liver tissue was more than fourfold higher, and there was still no sign of liver toxicity: bilirubin, serum glutamicoxaloacetic transaminase and serum glutamic pyruvic transaminase remained within the 5% and 95% range of the normal values during the entire follow-up period of 35 days. Unfortunately, at higher L-PAM doses in the IHP the rats died due to systemic toxicity, probably related to redistribution of L-PAM from saturated liver tissue to the bloodstream after the washout and termination of isolation. The concentration of L-PAM in tumor tissue was almost four times higher in the IHP-treated rats than in the rats treated with HAI. The tissue distribution of L-PAM therefore is remarkably different from that of MMC, which may be explained by the fact that L-PAM is actively transported into cells by an amino acid carrier system. The L-PAM concentration in liver and tumor tissue was significantly higher than in the perfusate and plasma.

As with MMC we studied the effects of L-PAM on tumor cell cycle kinetics and tumor growth. Garcia et al. (1988) showed a clear correlation between increasing concentrations of L-PAM and the number of DNA crosslinks. Tobey (1975) and Rao and Rao (1976) reported that the G_2 phase was most sensitive to DNA crosslinking. Several studies demonstrated that a transient block of tumor cells in G_2 phase at lower doses of L-PAM shifted to an irreversible S-phase block by increasing the dose. Progress from G_0/G_1 to S is affected last (Barlogie and Drewinko 1977). In our study HAI with the maximally tolerated dose (6 mg/kg) resulted in an accumulation of tumor cells in the late S and G_2/M phase, whereas IHP with 12 mg/kg resulted in blockage of tumor cells in G_0/G_1 and early S phases. These results suggest higher concentrations of L-PAM in the tumor cells following IHP, resulting in an increased number of DNA crosslinks. Vistica (1983) demonstrated that a small increase in the intracellular concentration of L-PAM (2–5 pmol/10^5 cells) markedly increases cytotoxicity. As might be expected from these findings, the antitumor effect of IHP was much greater than that of HAI with their respective maximally tolerated doses of L-PAM. All rats treated with IHP (12 mg/kg) showed complete remission (Fig. 3), whereas the tumors in rats treated with HAI (6 mg/kg) showed significant growth delay but a steady growth of all tumors.

Based on these rat studies and the fact that no hepatotoxicity was seen in patients treated with L-PAM 0.5 mg/kg in the IHP setting (Hafstrom et al. 1990) or after systemic treatment with a high dose of L-PAM (180 mg/m^2: five times higher than recommended for intravenous treatment) followed by autologous bone marrow transplantation (Lazarus et al. 1983), we started a phase I/II study with L-PAM 0.5 mg/kg in 1991.

Up to now we have treated 50 patients with L-PAM: 24 patients in a dose-finding study (0.5–4.0 mg/kg) and 26 patients in an ongoing phase II trial with a fixed dose of 200 mg L-PAM administrated as a bolus in the isolated circuit. In the first 21 L-PAM treated patients the same IHP technique (Fig. 2) was used as in the MMC trial. With this technique leakage of perfusate, as monitored with ^{99m}-Tc-labeled red blood cells, ranged from 0 to 30% and compromised the duration of IHP in up to 35% of the treated patients (maximally accepted leakage depended on total dose). In two patients leakage from the perfusion circuit to the systemic circulation unfortunately resulted in lethal leukopenia. In the one patient treated with L-PAM 4.0 mg/kg we observed lethal leukopenia plus serious hepatotoxic side effects. Therefore we consider 3.0 mg/kg to be the maximally tolerated dose of L-PAM in IHP in humans.

Because of the unacceptably high percentage of patients who could not be subjected to an entire hour of perfusion, the technique was changed as described above and depicted in Fig. 3. Since the change in technique 29 patients have been treated and in only two patients was the 1-h perfusion not completed because of leakage.

All patients were treated with granulocyte colony-stimulating factor (filgastim, or Neupogen) from the first day after perfusion until 1 day after the nadir of the white blood cellcount to prevent postoperative serious leukopenia. Until now, no hepatotoxic side effects were observed except for the patient treated with L-PAM 4.0 mg/kg.

Preliminary data from the phase I/II study suggest a relation between the dose of L-PAM and the tumor response. An objective partial response was observed on follow-up CT scans in five patients, and in one patient we found complete remission (still alive 49 months after IHP). The median survival of the patients treated during the phase I/II study was 18 months, which is comparable to the median survival in the group treated with MMC 30 mg/m^2.

Discussion

The principle of a steep dose–response curve has been well established in many experimental tumor models. To exploit the observed dose–response relation while maintaining tolerable systemic drug levels, hepatic artery infusion has been used in many clinical studies. The rationale of this approach rests on the observation of high hepatic extraction of selected drugs, allowing dose escalation. Furthermore, hepatic metastases derive most of their blood supply from the hepatic artery. In prospective randomized trials comparing systemic chemotherapy (5-fluorouracil or floxuridine) with HAI (floxuridine), significantly improved tumor responses were observed (Kemeny 1995; Vahrmeijer et al. 1995; Meta-Analysis Group in Cancer 1996), but the number of patients cured or with complete remission was limited, and the median survival was not significantly prolonged.

Isolated liver perfusion techniques have been developed by research groups to improve selective exposure of the target organ to still higher antitumor drug doses and concentrations so as to maximally exploit the dose–response relation (Skibba and Quebbeman 1986; van de Velde et al. 1986; Aigner et al. 1988; Hafstrom et al. 1994; Marinelli et al. 1996). We developed a reliable and technically feasible technique of IHP with a sensitive method for continuous leakage detection in pigs and a comparable technique in a rat colorectal cancer model. Twelve years after the first preclinical experiments we started a phase I/II study with MMC based on successful IHP with MMC in both pigs and rats. The clinical study, however, showed that MMC is too toxic for the liver cells and especially the liver vasculature. Four patients developed VOD. In one patient the VOD was subclinical and asymptomatic; in two patients it was symptomatic but not serious and reversible; and in one patient it was serious, with coagulopathy, encephalopathy, fluid overload, congestive heart failure, pulmonary insufficiency, renal failure, and portal hypertension with gastrointestinal bleeding resulting in death. For this reason we stopped perfusing livers with MMC and recommend MMC not be used in future clinical IHP studies.

We continued our IHP studies with a phase I/II study using L-PAM. As in the rat studies no hepatic toxicity was observed up to the maximally tolerated dose of 3.0 mg/kg. Dose-limiting toxicity was leukopenia even in patients with no leakage from the IHP circuit to the systemic circulation during the 1-h perfusion. Probably the leakage of intravascular L-PAM, the L-PAM redistribution (diffusion out of liver tissue), or both after termination of isolation causes the dose-limiting systemic toxicity despite a washout with 3.0 l of Haemaccel at the end of the perfusion.

During the dose-finding study the 1-h perfusion could not be completed in 35% of the patients due to leakage to the systemic circulation of the preoperatively determined maximally allowed amount of radiolabeled red blood cells. In most patients there was no other sign of leakage than decreased radioactivity in the isolated circuit and simultaneously increased radioactivity in the systemic circulation (no change in total volume in the isolated circuit, constant flow volume and pressure, hemodynamically stable patient). Leakage was later confirmed by the increased L-PAM concentration in the plasma samples collected during perfusion according to protocol. For this reason we recommend use of a leakage detection system even if, from a surgical point of view, technically perfect perfusion is being performed. We feel confident with our leakage detection system, but perhaps using radiolabeled albumin instead of radiolabeled red blood cells is even better.

To improve leakage control we changed the perfusion technique in humans (Fig. 3). Since the changes in technique, as described above only 2 of 29 treated patients have not completed 1 h of perfusion. Probably the double-lumen catheter interfered with unimpeded outflow of hepatic venous blood into the intrahepatic caval vein, requiring higher intrahepatic and intracaval pressure and promoting leakage to the systemic circulation whenever there is a minimal leak.

Although the phase II study with fixed-dose L-PAM (200 mg) has not been completed (patients are still entering the study), we already know that the number of complete remissions is limited. Perhaps the median survival will be better than in the phase I/II studies with MMC and L-PAM, but it will not be dramatically improved.

To further improve tumor response and patient survival, the possibilities with L-PAM during IHP must be exploited further in combination with hyperthermia followed by adjuvant treatment modalities that eliminate or control residual disease. The rationale for IHP under mild hyperthermia is that it enhances the cytotoxic activity of the anticancer agent L-PAM and has cytotoxic effects of its own (Bates and Mackillop 1990). These new strategies should be studied in proper phase I/II (multicenter) trials.

References

Ackerman NB, Lien WM, Kondi ES, Silverman NA (1969) The blood supply of experimental liver metastases. I. The distribution of hepatic artery and portal vein blood to "small" and "large" tumors. Surgery 66:1067–1072

Aigner KR, Walther H, Link KH (1988) Isolated liver perfusion with MMC/5-FU: surgical technique, pharmacokinetics, clinical results. Contrib Oncol 29:229–246

Barlogie B, Drewinko B (1977) Lethal and kinetic response of cultured human lymphoid cells to melphalan. Cancer Treat Rep 61:425–436

Bates DA, Mackillop WJ (1990) The effect of hyperthermia in combination with melphalan on drug-sensitive and drug-resistant CHO cells in vitro. Br J Cancer 62:183–188

Crooke ST, Bradner WT (1976) Mitomycin C: a review. Cancer Treat Rev 3:121–139

De Brauw LM, Marinelli A, van de Velde CJ, Hermans J, Tjaden UR, Erkelens C, de Bruijn EA (1991) Pharmacological evaluation of experimental isolated liver perfusion and hepatic artery infusion with 5-fluorouracil. Cancer Res 51:1694–1700

Doll DC, Weiss RB, Issell BF (1985) Mitomycin: ten years after approval for marketing. J Clin Oncol 276–286

Dorr RT, Bowden GT, Alberts DS, Liddil JD (1985) Interactions of mitomycin C with mammalian DNA detected by alkaline elution. Cancer Res 45:3510–3516

Garcia ST, McQuillan A, Panasci L (1988) Correlation between the cytotoxicity of melphalan and DNA crosslinks as detected by the ethidium bromide fluorescence assay in the F1 variant of B16 melanoma cells. Biochem Pharmacol 37:3189–3192

Gottfried MR, Sudilovsky O (1982) Hepatic veno-occlusive disease after high-dose mitomycin C and autologous bone marrow transplantation therapy. Hum Pathol 13:646–650

Hafstrom LR, Rudenstam C, Holmberg SB, Schersten TS, Ehrsson H (1990) The pharmacokinetics of melphalan in regional hyperthermic liver perfusion. Reg Cancer Treat 3:23–26

Hafstrom LR, Holmberg SB, Naredi PL, Lindner PG, Bengtsson A, Tidebrant G, Schersten TS (1994) Isolated hyperthermic liver perfusion with chemotherapy for liver malignancy. Surg Oncol 3:103–108

Kemeny NE (1995) Regional chemotherapy of colorectal cancer. Eur J Cancer 31A:1271–1276

Kemeny NE, Conti JA, Cohen A, Campana P, Huang Y, Shi WJ, Botet J, Pulliam S, Bertino JR (1994) Phase II study of hepatic arterial floxuridine, leucovorin, and dexamethasone for unresectable liver metastases from colorectal carcinoma. J Clin Oncol 12:2288–2295

Lazarus HM, Gottfried MR, Herzig RH, Phillips GL, Weiner RS, Sarna GP, Fay J, Wolff SN, Sudilovsky O, Gale RP, Herzig GP (1982) Veno-occlusive disease of the liver after high-dose mitomycin C therapy and autologous bone marrow transplantation. Cancer 49:1789–1795

Lazarus HM, Herzig RH, Graham Pole J, Wolff SN, Phillips GL, Strandjord S, Hurd D, Forman W, Gordon EM, Coccia P et al (1983) Intensive melphalan chemotherapy and cryopreserved autologous bone marrow transplantation for the treatment of refractory cancer. J Clin Oncol 1:359–367

Marinelli A, Dijkstra FR, van Dierendonck JH, Kuppen PJ, Cornelisse CJ, van de Velde CJ (1991a) Effectiveness of isolated liver perfusion with mitomycin C in the treatment of liver tumours of rat colorectal cancer. Br J Cancer 64:74–78

Marinelli A, Pons DH, Vreeken JA, Nagesser SK, Kuppen PJ, Tjaden UR, van de Velde CJ (1991b) High mitomycin C concentration in tumour tissue can be achieved by isolated liver perfusion in rats. Cancer Chemother Pharmacol 28:109–114

Marinelli A, van Dierendonck JH, van Brakel GM, Irth H, Kuppen PJ, Tjaden UR, van de Velde CJ (1991c) Increasing the effective concentration of melphalan in experimental rat liver tumours: comparison of isolated liver perfusion and hepatic artery infusion. Br J Cancer 64:1069–1075

Marinelli A, de Brauw LM, Beerman H (1996) Isolated liver perfusion with mitomycin C in the treatment of colorectal cancer metastases confined to the liver. Jpn J Clin Oncol 26:341–350

Marquet RL, Westbroek DL, Jeekel J (1984) Interferon treatment of a transplantable rat colon adenocarcinoma: importance of tumor site. Int J Cancer 33:689–692

Meta-Analysis Group in Cancer (1996) Reappraisal of hepatic arterial infusion in the treatment of nonresectable liver metastases from colorectal cancer. J Natl Cancer Inst 88:252–258

Rao AP, Rao PN (1976) The cause of G_2-arrest in Chinese hamster ovary cells treated with anticancer drugs. J Natl Cancer Inst 57:1139–1143

Runia RD, de Brauw LM, Kothuis BJ, Pauwels EK, van de Velde CJ (1987) Continuous measurement of leakage during isolated liver perfusion with a radiotracer. Int J Rad Appl Instrum [B] 14:113–118

Shulman HM, McDonald GB, Matthews D, Doney KC, Kopecky KJ, Gauvreau JM, Thomas ED (1980) An analysis of hepatic venocclusive disease and centrilobular hepatic degeneration following bone marrow transplantation. Gastroenterology 79:1178–1191

Skibba JL, Quebbeman EJ (1986) Tumoricidal effects and patient survival after hyperthermic liver perfusion. Arch Surg 121:1266–1271

Sobrero AF, Aschele C, Bertino JR (1997) Fluorouracil in colorectal cancer – a tale of two drugs: implications for biochemical modulation. J Clin Oncol 15:368–381

Tobey RA (1975) Different drugs arrest cells at a number of distinct stages in G_2. Nature 254:245–247

Vahrmeijer AL, van Dierendonck JH, van de Velde CJ (1995) Treatment of colorectal cancer metastases confined to the liver. Eur J Cancer 31A:1238–1242

Van de Velde CJ, Kothuis BJ, Barenbrug HW, Jongejan N, Runia RD, de Brauw LM, Zwaveling A (1986) A successful technique of in vivo isolated liver perfusion in pigs. J Surg Res 41:593–599

Van Ooijen B, Wiggers T, Meijer S, van der Heijde MN, Slooff MJ, van de Velde CJ, Obertop H, Gouma DJ, Bruggink ED, Lange JF et al (1992) Hepatic resections for colorectal metastases in The Netherlands: a multiinstitutional 10-year study. Cancer 70:28–34

Vistica DT (1983) Cellular pharmacokinetics of the phenylalanine mustards. Pharmacol Ther 22:379–406

Wanebo HJ, Semoglun C, Attiyeh F, Stearns MJ Jr (1978) Surgical management of patients with primary operable colorectal cancer and synchronous liver metastases. Am J Surg 135:81–85

Wang LQ, Persson BG, Bergqvist L, Bengmark S (1994) Influence of dearterialization on distribution of absolute tumor blood flow between hepatic artery and portal vein. Cancer 74:2454–2459

IV. Tumor Necrosis Factor

Molecular Mechanisms of TNF Receptor-Mediated Signaling

N. P. Malek, J. Pluempe, S. Kubicka, M. P. Manns, and C. Trautwein[1]

Department of Gastroenterology and Hepatology, Medizinische Hochschule Hannover, D-30623 Hannover, Germany
([1] Address for Correspondence)

Abstract

Tumor necrosis factor *α* (TNF*α*) is a proinflammatory cytokine involved in a variety of physiological and pathological conditions. During the past several years substantial progress has been made toward a better understanding of how a single cytokine is able to exert obviously opposing effects (e.g., apoptosis and growth). This review focuses on the recently discovered TNF-receptor (TNFR)-associated proteins involved in the activation of intracellular signal-transduction cascades. It explains which classes of proteins have been described so far and how these factors are able to mediate different biological functions after TNFR activation.

Introduction

Tumor necrosis factor *α* (TNF*α*) is a cytokine produced by activated macrophages and in smaller amounts by several other cell types. After its isolation during the 1980s considerable efforts were made to understand the molecular mechanisms of its diverse biological effects (Aggarval et al. 1984; Pennica et al. 1984). The original interest was focused on the antitumoral activity in vitro and its ability to cause hemorrhagic necrosis in transplanted tumors in vivo (Carswell et al. 1975). In addition to its activity against transformed cells, TNF*α* exerts various effects on some normal cell types (Dayer et al. 1985; Gamble et al. 1985), thereby implicating it as an important mediator in various physiological and pathophysiological conditions (i.e., septic shock, cerebral malaria, and others) (Beutler 1992).

During the past several years TNF*α* has been shown to be an important mediator of apoptosis (programmed cell death) (Kerr et al. 1972). Apoptosis is a reaction of mammalian cells induced by a variety of exogenous stimuli (e.g., the appearance or disappearance of cytokines and growth factors or changes in intercellular interactions). Apoptosis is now known to be one of the most important biological processes involved in the regulation of development, growth, and tumorigenesis (Tomei and Cope 1991, 1994; Williams

Recent Results in Cancer Research, Vol. 147

1991). Signals received from a cell's environment are interpreted in the context of internal information, such as cell type and developmental state (Williams and Smith 1993). Therefore exogenous factors reponsible for the decision toward self-destruction are often not exclusively involved in the control of apoptosis. The diversity of biological functions exerted by a cytokine such as TNFα can be explained by the simultaneous induction of intracellular signal transduction pathways necessary for the induction of apoptosis and the promotion of cell growth and differentiation. Therefore the TNF family of cell surface receptors (TNFRs) provides a model system of cytokine receptors involved in the control of various biological processes, especially the induction of pro- and antiapoptotic stimuli.

TNF Ligand and Receptor Families

The cytokine TNFα belongs to a family of nine known ligands – TNFα, lymphotoxin-α (LTα)/TNFβ, FAS-ligand (FasL), OX40L, CD40L, CD27L, CD30L, 4-1 BBL, and lymphotoxin-β that activate structurally related corresponding receptor proteins known as the TNFR superfamily (Smith et al. 1994). All ligand proteins consist of three identical polypeptide chains; only lymphotoxin-β is made up of two β- and one α-lymphotoxin subunit.

Although all ligands are class II membrane proteins defined by the location of the C-terminus within the extracellular space, they display not more than 20–25% homology at the protein level. The area of highest structural homology is located within a 150-amino-acid stretch at the C-terminus of the protein, the region that has been identified as the receptor-binding site. Although most TNF-related proteins function as multimeric membrane-bound factors that induce receptor aggregation, TNFα, LTα, and FasL are also functional in their soluble form.

So far 12 transmembrane proteins consisting of two identical subunits have been identified as members of the TNFR superfamily: TNF-R1 (p55), TNF-RII (p75), TNF-RP, FAS, OX-40, 4-1BB, CD40, CD30, CD27, poxvirus PV-T2, and PV-A53R gene products, and the p75 NGFR. The hallmark of this family of type I membrane receptor proteins is the presence of cysteine-rich amino acid motifs located in the extracellular ligand-binding domain of the receptor. These cysteine-rich domains (CRDs) are characterized by approximately 6 cysteine residues interspersed within a stretch of 40 amino acids. The functional importance of the CRDs lies in their capability to form interreceptor contacts, allowing formation of multimeric receptor complexes. Crystallographic studies of the extracellular domain of the 55-kD a TNF receptor in the absence of its ligand yield a dimeric protein arranged head-to-head to each other. The so-called molecular switch model has been developed from this observation. It is based on the hypothesis that a dimeric receptor protein is contacted by a trimeric ligand, leading to a rearrangement in the receptor's conformation that permits signal transduction through the activated receptor (reviewed by Smith et al. 1994).

Despite the membrane-bound multimeric protein complexes, soluble forms of TNF-RI, TNF-RII, CD40, CD30, CD27, 4-1BB, and Fas generated by proteolytic cleavage, or in the case of 4-1BB by alternative splicing, have been described. The physiological function of these soluble receptors is currently unknown.

TNFR-Associated Proteins

A common mechanism of signal transduction by cytokine or growth factor receptors is the tyrosine phosphorylation of downstream signal-transducing proteins, activating signaling cascades, which finally lead to the initiation or repression of gene expression. A striking feature of TNFR-I and TNFR-II is the lack of any domains within their intracellular regions able to exert catalytical activity. Therefore receptor-associated proteins were thought to function as the transducers in TNF-induced signaling (Tartaglia and Goeddel 1992; Beyaert and Fiers 1994).

The search for such molecules resulted in identification of the TNFR-associated factors 1 and 2 (TRAF-1 and TRAF-2) (Rothe et al. 1994). The common characteristic of TRAF proteins is the so-called TRAF domain at the protein *C*-terminus (Fig. 1). It is further divided into two subdomains in which the *C*-terminal subdomain seems to be specific for TRAF proteins and responsible for the TNFR association. The more *N*-terminal part, which is less conserved, forms a coiled-coil α-helix motif known to be involved in protein oligomerization. TRAF-2/TRAF-1 heterodimers and TRAF-2 homodimers are able to bind the *C*-terminal part of TNFR-II, which is responsible for signal transduction. Altogether 78 amino acids at the *C*-terminal, intracellular domain of TNFR-II are responsible for the detected NF-κB activation after ligand crosslinking. Overexpression of TRAF-2 also leads to activation of NF-κB, whereas deletion of the *N*-terminal RING-finger domain (Freemont 1993), believed to enable

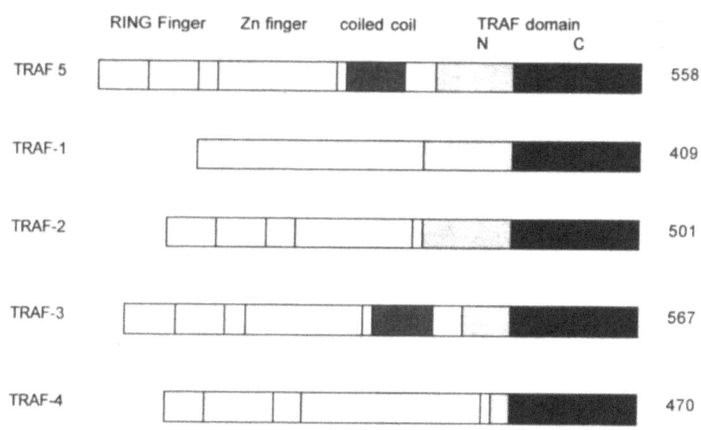

Fig. 1. Structural domains of the TRAF protein family

protein DNA and protein–protein interactions by the formation of two zinc finger structures, abolishes this function (Rothe et al. 1995b; Hsu et al. 1996). These results lead to a model of TNFR-II-induced activation of downstream effector proteins in which homo- or heterodimerized TRAF-2 proteins are linked to TNFR-II via their *C*-terminal TRAF domains, whereas signal transduction is mediated by the *N*-terminal RING-finger motif.

TRAF-5 is a 64-kDa protein cloned in the search for TRAF homologues using degenerated primers corresponding to the conserved TRAF regions of TRAF-1, TRAF-2, and TRAF-3. Overexpression in embryonic kidney cells led to the activation of NF-κB, revealing a strong functional similarity with TRAF-2. In contrast with TRAF-2, co-immunoprecipitation experiments demonstrated the formation of complexes between the lymphotoxin β-receptor (LT-βR) and TRAF-5, implicating the protein in signaling mediated by the LT-βR (Cheng et al. 1995; Nakano et al. 1996).

The 62-kDa TRAF-3 protein (CRAF-1, CAP-1, CD40bp, LAP-1) is another recently identified member of the TRAF family. At the protein level it is most closely related to TRAF-2 but differs from this protein by the existence of an isoleucine zipper (Landschulz et al. 1988) located between the *N*-terminal RING and zinc finger and the *C*-terminal TRAF domain. Interactions of TRAF-3 with TNFR-I and TNFR-II have been described, but the protein seems mainly be involved in CD40 receptor-induced signaling. Furthermore, overexpression of TRAF-3 can suppress TNFR-II and CD40-induced NF-κB activation, suggesting that TRAF-3 plays a role in the negative regulation of protein activation and gene expression.

The recently discovered TRAF-6 protein extends the role of TRAF proteins of being signal transducers of the TNFR superfamily. Although structurally related to the other TRAF proteins, TRAF-6 is not involved in TNF but interleukin-1 (IL-1)-induced signaling. Furthermore, after IL-1 treatment the protein interacts with a receptor-associated tyrosine kinase (IRAK), thereby connecting the kinase to the downstream signaling cascade, leading to the activation of NF-κB (Cao et al. 1996). Another protein involved in the regulation of downstream signal transduction events mediated by TRAF proteins, named TRAF-interacting protein (TRIP) has been cloned. This protein is able to associate with the TNFR-2 or CD30 signaling complex through its interaction with TRAF-2, thereby inhibiting the activation of NF-κB (Lee et al. 1997). In contrast, members of the C-IAP (cellular inhibitor of apoptosis) family have been shown to inhibit apoptosis induced by TNF. The proteins contain a *C*-terminal RING finger and *N*-terminal baculovirus IAP repeat (BIR) motifs with which they associate with TRAF-1/TRAF-2 heterodimers. Unlike TRIP, c-IAP proteins do not inhibit NF-κB activation; rather, they have been implicated in the inhibition of cell death (Rothe et al. 1995a; Duckett et al. 1996; Liston et al. 1996). Obviously the TRAF family of receptor-associated proteins offers a possibility of mediating opposing effects (i.e., cell activation/growth or cell death in response to TNFR activation). Which type of signal transducer (c-IAPs or TRIP) is recruited to the TNFR seems to be determined by their availability and by the presence of various TRAF proteins.

As activation of NF-κB is a common feature of various TRAF proteins, overexpression of TRAF-2 also leads to the induction of SAPK/JNK activity (Natoli et al. 1997; Reinhard et al. 1997). Activation of this kinase is part of the cellular stress-response system, known to be activated by various exogenous stimuli (e.g., ultraviolet irradiation, protein synthesis inhibitors, and TNFα). By using a dominant negative TRAF-2 mutant, lacking the *N*-terminal RING finger domain, the TNFα-induced activation of JNK can be completely blocked, whereas other inducers of the stress-activated kinase pathway are not affected in regard to their capability to stimulate kinase activity (Liu et al. 1996). The physiological role of the SAPK/JNK cascade activation has not been thoroughly defined. However, SAPK/JNK activity is required for the induction of apoptosis in growth factor-deprived sympathetic neurons as well as in fibroblasts and leukemia cells (Xia et al. 1995; Verheij et al. 1996).

Death Domain Proteins

The death domain is a conserved protein–protein interraction motif of about 80 amino acids, first identified in the intracellular *C*-terminal regions of TNFR-1 and the FAS receptor (Tartaglia et al. 1993). This region is sufficient to induce signals for apoptosis, antiviral activity, activation of an acidic sphingomyelinase, and (in conjunction with residues in the *N*-terminal portion) induction of nitric oxide (NO) synthase activity (Tartaglia et al. 1993). However, the lack of catalytic activity within the intracellular portion of the TNFR-1 led to the hypothesis that, as with TNFR-2-mediated signaling, interacting proteins might be the transducers of the death signal activated after ligand binding.

Using the yeast two-hybrid system, a novel gene product, the TNFR-1-associated death domain protein (TRADD), has been cloned. The 34.2-kDa TRADD protein was found in all tissues examined, although its expression level was relatively low. Interaction with TNFR-1 was shown to be mediated by a *C*-terminal 111-amino-acid death domain, 23% identical to the death domain of the TNFR-1. Overexpression of TRADD leads to the induction of apoptosis, resembling a phenotype observed in cells overexpressing TNFR-1. However, the apoptotic process could be inhibited by CrmA, a protein derived from the cowpox virus, that is able to prevent the pro-apoptotic action of the ICE and ICE-like proteases (Hsu et al. 1995). Deletion mutagenesis studies identified the death domain of TRADD as being responsible for TNFR-1 binding, NF-κB activation, and the induction of apoptosis.

Interestingly, TRADD is unable to associate with the death domain of the FAS receptor, demonstrating the uniqueness and individuality of each receptor despite the presence of a death domain. Although TRADD does not associate with the FAS receptors, death domain, a protein called FADD (FAS-associated protein with death domain) also designated MORT-1, is responsible for the induction of apoptosis by the FAS receptor. Like TRADD, the 23.3-kDa FADD protein is ubiquitously expressed and highly selective in its strong association with the FAS receptor (Boldin et al. 1995; Chinnaiyan et al. 1995). Unlike TRADD, the death domain of FADD is not required for the induction of apoptosis; instead, a discrete *N*-terminal region – the death effector domain – proved to be necessary.

Surprisingly, a yeast two-hybrid screen identified a strong interaction between the FADD and TRADD proteins. During the same search, TRAF-2 was identified as being able to associate with TRADD. Deletion mutagenesis analysis revealed that the interaction between TRADD and FADD is mediated via the *C*-terminal death domains of TRADD and FADD, whereas the *N*-terminus of TRADD associates with the *C*-terminal TRAF domain of TRAF-2. Functional analysis using dominant negative mutants of FADD and TRAF-2 showed that the interaction with FADD is necessary for the induction of apoptosis, and the association with TRAF-2 induced NF-κB activation (Hsu et al. 1996). Identification of TRADD as an adaptor protein able to recruit TRAF-2 and FADD to the TNFR-1 offered a molecular mechanism for the question of how TNF might be able to exert different functions, such as induction of apoptosis and activation of NF-κB (Fig. 2).

Downstream Effector Mechanisms

Identification of TNFR-associated proteins and the observation that overexpression of these proteins leads to apoptosis and activation of NF-κB/JNK were important steps toward understanding TNF-mediated signaling. How activation of the cell death machinery, including the ICE proteases, and the induction of signal transduction cascades is generated by these protein-complexes is nevertheless not known.

By using nanoelectrospray tandem mass spectrometry and the yeast two-hybrid interaction cloning approach, a new protein able to interact with the FAS death-inducing signaling complex (DISC) and FADD in a ligand-dependent manner has been cloned (Boldin et al. 1996; Muzio et al. 1996). Sequence analysis showed that the new protein, named FLICE/MACH/caspase 8, encoded a member of the ICE protease family, characterized by a *C*-terminal 260-amino-acid region of strong homology with other known ICE-related cysteine proteases. In addition it contains two *N*-terminal tandem regions of homology with the death effector domain of FADD through which it interacts with this receptor-associated protein. Moreover, a dominant negative form blocked TNF- and FAS-induced apoptosis, emphasizing its role in both signaling pathways.

Although TNF is able to induce apoptosis in diseased cells (transformed or infected by viruses) and cells treated with protein synthesis inhibitors, normal cells are largely unaffected by TNF treatment (Beyaert and Fiers 1994). This phenomenon is expanded by the observation that pretreatment with TNF protects cells from the suicidal mechanisms induced by TNF and protein synthesis inhibitors applied in parallel. Therefore TNF can induce protective proteins (Wong and Goeddel 1988), allowing a cell to survive TNF

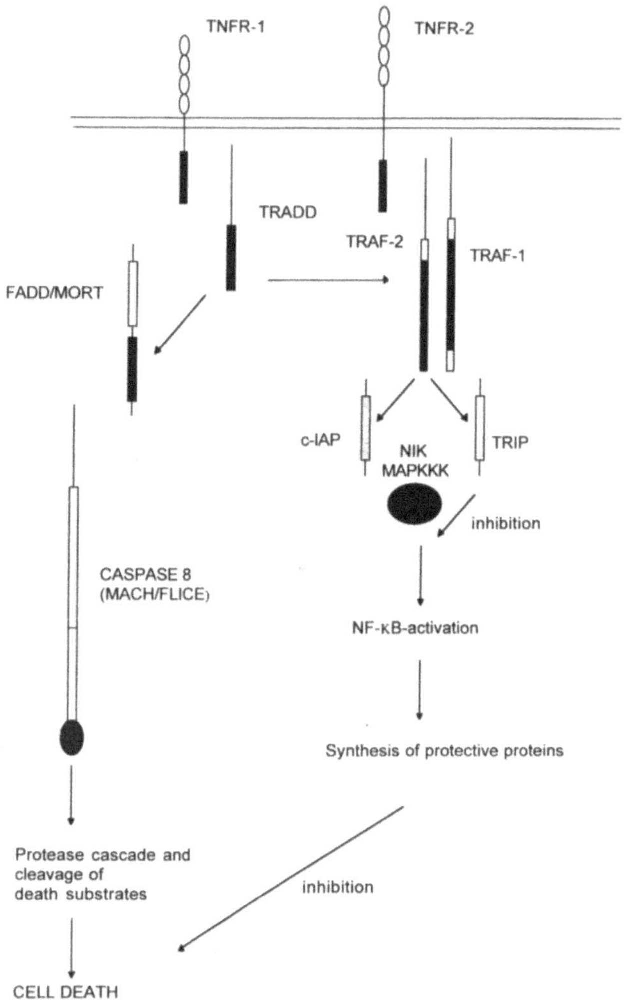

Fig. 2. Proteins involved in TNFR-1 and TNFR-2 signal transduction

cytotoxicity when combined with a protein synthesis inhibitor. The transcription factor NF-κB has been identified as being a potential mediator of these TNF-induced protective mechanisms (Beg and Baltimore 1996; Van Antwerp et al. 1996; Wang et al. 1996). Activation of NF-κB by cytokines such as TNF and IL-1 is mediated via phosphorylation of its cytoplasmic inhibitor proteins (collectively called IκB), leading to the ubiquitination of this inhibitor, thereby targeting it for degradation by the proteolytic enzymes. Overexpression of the NF-κB p65 (ReIA) subunit increased the cells' ability to survive TNF cytotoxicity, while blocking NF-κB activation by use of a dominant negative form of IκB or by agents that chemically inhibit NF-κB activation; it significantly induced apoptosis of the treated cells (Wu et al. 1996). Furthermore cell lines derived from p65 knockout mice exhibited dramatically decreased viability after TNF treatment (Beg and Baltimore 1996).

The exact mechanism by which NF-κB is activated, i.e., the kinase(s) responsible for IκB phosphorylation, are not known. The induction of NF-κB by TNF involves the above-described association of the adaptor protein TRADD with the TNFR-associated protein TRAF-2. A recently identified serine/threonine kinase, NIK, is able to bind TRAF-2 and activate NF-κB after overexpression, leading to markedly increased resistance to TNF cytotoxicity. NIK shows high sequence homology with kinases that act within the mitogen-activated protein (MAP) kinase cascade, such as MAP kinase kinase kinase, and might function in a similar manner (Malinin et al. 1997). The identification of NF-κB as being a TNF-induced antiapoptotic protein obviously explains why TNF in conjunction with protein synthesis inhibitors exerts the observed cytotoxic effects. By blocking protein synthesis, NF-κB is unable to induce the production of protective proteins, thereby enabling the FADD-activated suicide machinery to execute its deadly program. Cell lines derived from $p65^{-/-}$ mice are viable but exhibit markedly increased sensitivity against TNF, confirming the phenotype of a $p65^{-/-}$ mouse that died prenatally by massive apoptosis of the liver (Beg et al. 1995; Beg and Baltimore 1996). In contrast, results obtained from experiments employing various inhibitors of NF-κB activation, which on their own lead to apoptotic destruction of the treated cells, argue for a not exclusively TNF-dependent mechanism of NF-κB protection (Wu et al. 1996).

During the last several years much progress has been made toward a better understanding of how TNF exerts its pleiotropic functions. The identification of different receptor-associated proteins able to induce pro- and antiapoptotic functions explained many of the effects observed since the discovery of this cytokine. However, little is known about how the balance between the opposing processes is regulated. Which other factors and signaling cascades might be involved in this highly regulated framework? What are the downstream substrates of the caspases induced by TNF, and what are the main proteins activated by NF-κB to protect cells from their endogenous suicide program? Answering these so far unresolved questions might lead to a better understanding of how inflammatory and proliferative diseases can be treated by interfering with the molecular processes induced by TNF.

References

Aggarwal BB, Moffat B, Harkins RN (1984) Human lymphotoxin: production by a lymphoblastoid cell line: purification, and initial characterisation. J Biol Chem 259:686–691

Beg AA, Baltimore D (1996) An essential role for NF-κB in preventing TNFα induced cell death. Science 274:782–784

Beg AA, Sha WC, Bronson RT, Ghosh S, Baltimore D (1995) Embryonic lethality and liver degeneration in mice lacking the RelA component of NF-κB. Nature 376:167–170

Beutler B (ed) (1992) Tumor necrosis factor: the molecules and their emerging role in medicine. Raven, New York

Beyaert R, Fiers W (1994) Molecular mechanisms of tumor necrosis factor-induced cytotoxicity: FEBS Lett 340:9–16

Boldin MP, Varfolomeev EE, Pancer Z, Mett IL, Camonis JH, Wallach D (1995) A novel protein that interacts with the death domain of Fas/APO1 contains a sequence motif related to the death domain. J Biol Chem 270:7795–7798

Boldin MP, Goncharov TM, Golstev YV, Wallach D (1996) Involvement of MACH, a novel MORT1/FADD-interacting protease in Fas/APO-1 and TNF receptor induced cell death. Cell 81:803–815

Cao Z, Xiong J, Takeuchi M, Kurama T, Goeddel DV (1996) TRAF6 is a signal transducer for interleukin-1. Nature 383:443–446

Carswell EA, Old LJ, Kassel RL, Green S, Fiore N, Williamson B (1975) An endotoxin-induced serum factor that causes necrosis of tumors. Proc Natl Acad Sci USA 72:3666–3670

Cheng G, Cleary AM, Ye Z, Hong DI, Lederman S, Baltimore D (1995) Involvement of CRAF2, a relative of TRAF, in CD40 signalling. Science 267:1494–1498

Chinnaiyan AM, O'Rourke K, Tewari M, Dixit VM (1995) Fadd, a novel death domain-containing protein, interacts with the death domain of Fas and initiates apoptosis. Cell 81:505–512

Dayer JM, Beutler B, Cerami A (1985) Cachectin/tumor necrosis factor stimulates collagenase and prostaglandin E_2 production by human synovial cells and dermal fibroblasts. J Exp Med 162:2163–2168

Duckett CS, Nava VE, Gedrich RW, Clem RJ, Van Dongen JL, Gilfillan MC, Shiels H, Hardwick JM, Thompson CB (1996) A conserved family of cellular genes related to the baculovirus IAP gene encoding apoptosis inhibitors. EMBO J 15:2685–2694

Freemont PS (1993) The RING finger: a novel protein sequence motif related to the zinc finger. Ann NY Acad Sci 684:174–192

Gamble JR, Harlan JM, Klebanoff SJ, Vadas MA (1985) Stimulation of the adherence of neutrophils to umbilical vein endothelium by the human recombinant tumor necrosis factor. Proc Natl Acad Sci USA 82:8667–8671

Hsu H, Xiong J, Goeddel DV (1995) The TNF receptor 1-associated protein TRADD signals cell death and NF-κB activation. Cell 81:495–504

Hsu H, Shu HB, Pan MG, Goeddel DV (1996) TRADD-TRAF2 and TRADD–FADD interactions define two distinct TNF receptor 1 signal transduction pathways. Cell 84:299–308

Kerr JFR, Wyllie AH, Curie AR (1972) Apoptosis: a basic biological phenomenon with wide-ranging implications in tissue kinetics. Br J Cancer 26:239–257

Landschulz WH, Johnson PF, McKnight SL (1988) The leucine zipper: a hypothetical structure common to a new class of DNA binding proteins. Science 240:1759–1764

Lee SY, Lee SY, Choi Y (1997) TRAF-interacting protein (TRIP): a novel component of the tumor necrosis factor receptor (TNFR)- and CD30-TRAF signaling complexes that inhibits TRAF2-mediated NF-κB activation. J Exp Med 185:1275–1285

Liston P, Roy N, Tamai C, Lefevre C, Baird S, Cherton-Horvat G, Farahani R, McLean M, Ikeda JE, MacKenzie A, Korneluk RG (1996) Suppression of apoptosis in mammalian cells by NAIP and a related family of IAP genes. Nature 379:349–353

Liu ZG, Hsu H, Goeddel DV, Karin M (1996) Dissection of TNF receptor 1 effector functions: JNK activation is not linked to apoptosis while NF-κB activation prevents cell death. Cell 87:565–576

Malinin NL, Boldin MP, Kovalenko AV, Wallach D (1997) MAP3K-related kinase involved in NF-κB induction by TNF, CD95 and IL-1. Nature 385:540–544

Muzio M, Chinnaiyan AM, Kischkel FC, O'Rourke K, Shevchenko A, Ni J, Scaffidi C, Brentz JD, Zhang M, Gentz R et al (1996) FLICE a novel FADD homologous ICE/CED-3-like protease, is recruited to the CD95 (Fas/APO-1) death inducing signalling complex. Cell 85:817–827

Nakano H, Oshima H, Chung W, Williams-Abbott L, Ware CF, Yagita H, Okumura K (1996) TRAF5 an activator of NF-κB and putative signal transducer for the lymphotoxin-β receptor J Biol Chem 271:14661–14664

Natoli G, Costanzo A, Ianni A, Templeton DJ, Woodgett JR, Balsano C, Levrero M (1997) Activation of SAPK/JNK by a noncytotoxic TRAF2-dependent pathway. Science 275:200–203

Pennica D, Nedwin GE, Hayflick JS et al (1984) Human tumor necrosis factor: precursor structure, expression and homology to lymphotoxin. Nature 312:724–729

Reinhard C, Shamoon B, Venkatakrishna S, Williams L (1997) Tumor necrosis factor induced activation of c-jun N-terminal kinase is mediated by TRAF2. EMBO J 16:1080–1092

Rothe M, Wong SC, Henzel WJ, Goeddel DV (1994) A novel family of putative signal transducers associated with the cytoplasmic domain of the 75 kDa tumor necrosis factor receptor. Cell 78:681–692

Rothe M, Pan MG, Henzel WJ, Ares TM, Goeddel DV (1995a) The TNFR2-TRAF signaling complex contains two novel proteins related to baculoviral inhibitor of apoptosis proteins. Cell 83:1243–1252

Rothe M, Sarma V, Dixit VM, Goeddel DV (1995b) TRAF2 mediated activation of NF-κB by TNF receptor 2 and CD40. Science 269:1424–1427

Smith CA, Farrah T, Goodwin RG (1994) The TNF receptor superfamily of cellular and viral proteins: activation, costimulation, and death. Cell 76: 959–962

Tartaglia LA, Goeddel DV (1992) Two TNF receptors. Immunol Today 13:151–153

Tartaglia LA, Ayres TM, Wong GHW, Goeddel DV (1993) A novel domain within the 55 kDa TNF receptor signals cell death. Cell 74: 845–853

Tomei LD, Cope FO (1991) Apoptosis: the molecular basis of cell death. Cold Spring Harbor Laboratory, Cold Spring Harbor, NY

Tomei LD, Cope FO (1994) Apoptosis II: the molecular basis of apoptosis in disease. Cold Spring Harbor Laboratory, Cold Spring Harbor, NY

Van Antwerp DJ, Martin SJ, Kafri T, Green DR, Verma IM (1996) Suppression of TNFα induced apoptosis by NF-κB. Science 274:787–789

Verheij M, Bose R, Lin XH, Yao B, Jarvis WD, Grant S, Birrer MJ, Szabo E, Zon LI, Kyriakis JM, Halmovitz-Friedman A, Fuks Z, Kolesnick R (1996) Requirement for ceramide initiated SAPK/JNK signalling in stress induced apoptosis. Nature 380:75–79

Wang CY, Mayo MW, Baldwin JAS (1996) TNF and cancer therapy-induced apoptosis: potentiation by inhibition of NF-κB. Science 274:784–787

Williams GT (1991) Programmed cell death: apoptosis and oncogenesis. Cell 65:1097–1098

Williams GT, Smith CA (1993) Molecular regulation of apoptosis: genetic controls on cell death. Cell 74:777–779

Wong GHW, Goeddel DV (1988) Induction of manganous superoxide dismutase by tumor necrosis factor: possible protective mechanism. Science 242:941–944

Wu M, Lee H, Bellas RE, Schauer SL, Arsura M, Katz D, FitzGerald M, Rothstein TL, Sherr DH, Sonenshein GE (1996) Inhibition of NF-κB/Rel induces apoptosis of murine B cells. EMBO J 15:4682–4690

Xia Z, Dickens M, Raingeaud J, Davis RJ, Greenberg ME (1995) Opposing effects of ERK and JNK-p38 MAP kinases on apoptosis. Science 270:1326–1331

Isolated Hepatic Perfusion with Tumor Necrosis Factor *α* and Melphalan: Experimental Studies in Pigs and Phase I Data from Humans

M.R. de Vries[1], I.H. Borel Rinkes[1], C.J.H. van de Velde[2], T. Wiggers[1], R.A.E.M. Tollenaar[2], P.J.K. Kuppen[2], A.L. Vahrmeijer[2], and A.M.M. Eggermont[1]

[1] Department of Surgical Oncology, Dr. Daniël den Hoed Cancer Center, University Hospital Rotterdam, PO Box 5201, NL-3008 AE Rotterdam, The Netherlands
[2] Department of Surgery, University Hospital Leiden, Leiden, The Netherlands

Abstract

We report our experience with isolated hepatic perfusion (IHP) with tumor necrosis factor (TNF) and melphalan in an experimental pig study and of a phase I study in humans. IHP was performed with inflow catheters in the hepatic artery and portal vein and an outflow catheter in the caval vein. An extracorporeal venovenous bypass was used. IHP consisted of a 60-min perfusion with hyperthermia (> 41 °C). For the pig protocol rhTNF*α* 50 µg/kg alone ($n=5$) or rhTNF*α* 50µg/kg plus melphalan 1 mg/kg ($n=3$) were added. In two control pigs no drugs were added. In the phase I study, patients received melphalan 1 mg/kg with 0.4 mg rhTNF*α* ($n=8$) or 0.8 mg rhTNF*α* ($n=1$). After the perfusion the liver was washed with Macrodex before vascular continuity was restored. All pigs but one survived the procedure. Systemic leakage was less than 0.02%. Transient, mild liver toxicity was seen in all pigs, including controls, as demonstrated by liver enzyme assays and histology. There was no significant hemodynamic, cardiopulmonary hemotological, or renal toxicity. In the phase I clinical study there was leakage in one patient (cumulative leakage 20%). There were three perioperative deaths (one possibly drug-related). All patients demonstrated significant hepatotoxicity. Survival ranged from 6 to 26 months (median 10.3 months). All patients demonstrated a tumor response (partial response 5/6, 1/6 stable disease) with a median duration of 18 weeks. In contrast to our pig program, many problems were encountered in the phase I study. By using both the hepatic artery and portal vein for IHP we encountered more toxicity than expected based on data from the pig program, resulting in fatal coagulative disturbances in one patient who received the second rhTNF*α* dose. Furthermore, local control after one IHP with TNF*α* and melphalan is only temporary.

Introduction

The liver is the most common site of dissemination in patients with colorectal cancer, and if left untreated the median survival in these patients is ap-

Recent Results in Cancer Research, Vol. 147

proximately 6–9 months (Wagner et al. 1984). In contrast, 5-year survival rates as high as 35% have been reported for patients amenable to partial hepatic resection (Que and Nagorney 1994). Unfortunately, most colorectal metastases confined to the liver are not resectable (Genari 1992). Therefore it is mandatory to develop novel strategies to obtain tumor control in the liver.

Several techniques have been developed for regional therapy of hepatic malignancies, of which hepatic artery infusion (HAI) is most widely used (De Takats et al. 1994). Although HAI has been shown to improve short-term tumor response rates compared to systemic chemotherapy, it hardly affects survival, and significant dose-limiting toxicity has been encountered (De Takats et al. 1994).

Alternatively, isolated hepatic perfusion (IHP) with total vascular isolation of the liver in rats significantly increased intrahepatic drug concentrations when compared with HAI while maintaining sufficiently low systemic drug levels (Aigner 1988; De Brauw et al. 1988; Marinelli et al. 1991). With IHP hepatic rather than systemic toxicity may prove to be dose-limiting. Incidental clinical reports on IHP are promising, indicating the potential use of this technique in humans (Aigner 1988). It is clear that optimization of the IHP methodology is needed. In addition, it is presently unknown which drug(s) would provide optimal antitumor activity in the IHP setting.

A promising drug with important in vitro and in vivo antitumor effects is tumor necrosis factor α (TNFα), a cytokine produced mainly by activated macrophages (Carswell et al. 1975). In human systemic administration of TNFα in many phase I and II studies has resulted in considerable dose-limiting toxicity with dose levels at which no antitumor activity was observed (Feinberg et al. 1988; Spriggs et al. 1988). Multicenter studies have now shown that high-dose TNFα, in combination with the alkylating drug melphalan, can be used safely in isolated limb perfusion, where complete vascular isolation of the extremity involved ensures minimal systemic exposure to the drug (Lienard et al. 1992; Eggermont et al. 1996a, b). Although the exact mechanism of antitumor action by TNFα is unknown, endothelial injury of the tumor-associated vascular bed after IHP was ascribed to be essential in the genesis of tumor necrosis (Renard et al. 1994). Thus TNFα may be expected to prove effective against any histological tumor variant, provided the tumor has a well-developed vascular bed (Manusama et al. 1996).

It could be speculated that intrahepatic administration of TNFα induces significant hepatotoxicity, as Kupffer cells are known to release various cytokines in response to TNFα exposure (Busam et al. 1990). On the other hand, based on the synergy between TNFα and melphalan, considerable tumor responses could be anticipated. Therefore we first analyzed the effects of IHP with TNFα with and without melphalan, in pigs. For this purpose, a modification of the original IHP technique was developed and tested. Following this step we started a phase I clinical study in nine patients with colorectal metastases confined to the liver.

Materials and Methods

IHP Study in Pigs

In the IHP study in pigs, ten healthy pigs weighing 25–33 kg (median 30 kg) were used. All animals received humane care in compliance with our institution's guidelines on animal welfare. The IHP procedure has been described in detail elsewhere (Borel Rinkes et al. 1997).

In short, an arterial line, central venous catheter, and Swan-Ganz catheter were placed in all animals. The liver's vasculature was dissected free and isolated at a midline laparotomy. Following systemic heparinization, an extracorporeal venovenous bypass (VVB) circuit was created to shunt mesenteric, renal, and lower extremity blood around the liver to the heart. The VVB flow was aided by a passive centrifugal pump in a manner identical to the technique currently used during liver transplantation procedures. Next, the liver circuit was created by placing inflow catheters in the portal vein (PV) and hepatic artery (HA), and an outflow catheter in the infrahepatic vena cava inferior (VCI). These catheters were connected to a heart-lung machine, and the vascular isolation was completed by clamping the suprahepatic VCI and the suprarenal VCI. The liver was then perfused with a hyperthermic (>41 °C) perfusate consisting of a mixture of saline and erythrocytes. Once a stable perfusion was attained, the absence of systemic leakage from the IHP circuit was confirmed by injecting fluorescein into the arterial inflow port and illuminating the operative field with an ultraviolet (Woods) lamp.

After confirmation of total vascular isolation with no systemic leakage, the drugs were infused into the perfusion circuit. IHP consisted of a 60-min perfusion in five pigs with recombinant humane (rh) TNFα (50 μg/kg) alone and in three pigs with rhTNFα (50 μg/kg) plus melphalan (1 mg/kg). rhTNFα was administered as a bolus in the arterial line of the perfusion circuit; melphalan was given directly following rhTNFα bolus. In two control pigs no drugs were added (sham group). After a 60-min perfusion, the liver was washed thoroughly with a mixture of saline and Macrodex, decannulated, and vascular continuity restored. Pigs were observed for 4–6 weeks, whereafter they were sacrificed for macroscopic and histological evaluation.

Phase I Study

Study Design. The study was designed as a dose escalation study to assess the toxicity and maximal tolerated dose of rhTNFα in combination with melphalan (1 mg/kg body weight) in a hyperthermic, isolated hepatic perfusion. The study was performed in two centers: the University Hospital Rotterdam – Dr. Daniël den Hoed Cancer Center and the University Hospital Leiden. *Inclusion criteria* for IHP with TNFα and melphalan were (1) histological evidence of unresectable metastases of colorectal origin confined to the liver; (2) age between 18 and 70 years; and (3) Karnofsky performance status of

>80%. The *exclusion criteria* (summary) included (1) extrahepatic malignant disease; (2) > 50% hepatic tissue replacement by tumor; (3) liver cirrhosis; (4) signs of significant hepatic dysfunction [abnormal levels of aspartate aminotransferase (ASAT), alanine aminotransferase (ALAT), or alkaline phosphatase more than two times normal]; and (5) ascites or portal hypertension.

From January to June 1995, nine patients underwent IHP with TNFα and melphalan. All gave informed consent prior to treatment. The protocols were approved by the hospitals' ethics committees. There were six men and three women with a mean age of 59.8 years (range 49–65 years). The median replaced hepatic volume (RHV) was 20% (3.5–45.0%).

Operative Procedure and Leakage Monitoring. We used a technique similar to that in the pig study, as described above, with one adjustment. Once a stable counts-per-minute baseline was obtained from scintillation probes placed over the perfusate reservoir and VVB, 200 μCi ^{131}I-albumin was injected into the perfusate. Based on the systemic baseline count and the perfusion circuit volume, the percentage of leakage can be accurately calculated. If there was more than 1% leakage over 10 min, adjustments were made in the perfusion flow rates and cannula position in an attempt to identify the source of the leak prior to administering the rhTNFα and melphalan. The leak rate was monitored for the duration of the perfusion; and if the cumulative leak was more than 15%, the perfusion was halted and the perfusate flushed from the circuit. After the absence of leakage was confirmed, rhTNFα (0.4 mg in eight patients, 0.8 mg in one) was administered as a bolus in the arterial line of the perfusion circuit; melphalan (1 mg/kg) was given directly following the rhTNFα bolus. After a 60-min perfusion, the liver was washed thoroughly with a mixture of saline and Macrodex, decannulated, and the vascular continuity restored. Postoperatively the patients were monitored in the intensive care unit (ICU) for at least 48 h, primarily to evaluate for evidence of systemic toxicity due to rhTNFα.

Routine laboratory tests were performed once a day for the first week, at days 10, 14, 21, and 28, and every 2 months thereafter. True-cut biopsies of the liver and tumor tissues were performed before and during operation and 4–6 weeks after IHP. Tumor measurement was performed by computed tomographic (CT)-scan 2 and 4 weeks after IHP and every 2 months thereafter.

Drugs. Recombinant human TNFα (0.2 mg/ampoule) was a kind gift from Boehringer Ingelheim, Germany. The cytostatic drug melphalan (Alkeran) came as a sterile powder (100 mg) that was dissolved aseptically using solvent and diluent obtained from Burroughs Wellcome (London, UK).

Sampling Schedule. Blood samples were collected from a peripheral vein in siliconized 5-ml Vacutainer tubes (Becton Dickinson, Plymouth, UK) containing EDTA (10 nmol/l), soybean trypsin inhibitor (100 mg/l), and benzamidine (10 nmol/l) (Sigma Chemicals, Detroit, Mi, USA) to prevent in vitro activation. Samples were centrifuged immediately after collection at 5000 rpm for 5 min. Supernatant was stored at –70 °C until analysis.

The perfusate was sampled at 10-min intervals. Systemic plasma samples were collected on the day before ILP, during ILP at $t=0$, 30, and 60 min, and after perfusion (after release of the VCI clamp) at $t=1$, 5, 10, 20, 30, 60, 120, and 240 min, on days 1, 3, and 7, and thereafter weekly.

Assays. TNFα [normal value (N) < 5 pg/ml], secondary cytokines IL-6 (N < 10 pg/ml) and IL-8 (N < 20 pg/ml), and soluble TNF receptors [sTNFR-p55 (N < 2 ng/ml) and sTNFR-p75 (N < 2 ng/ml)] levels measured by enzyme-linked immunosorbent assay (ELISA) as described previously (Helle et al. 1991; Hack et al. 1992; Vreugdenhil et al. 1992 Leeuwenberg et al. 1994). The acute-phase proteins were measured by a nephelometric assay.

Coagulation and fibrinolysis were analyzed by measuring thrombin-antithrombin III (TAT) (N < 4 ng/ml), tissue type plasminogen activator (t-PA) (N < 2 ng/ml), and plasminogen activator inhibitor type I (PAI), (N < 30 ng/ml) by ELISA as described previously (Levi et al. 1992; De Boer et al. 1993), whereas plasmin-α_2-antiplasmin (PAP) (N < 7 nM) complexes were measured with a radioimmunoassay (RIA).

Histology. Multiple liver biopsies were performed before and directly following IHP and 4–6 weeks after IHP. The tissue samples were prepared for hemoatoxylin and eosin (HEE) staining and electron microscopy.

Statistics. Results are expressed as the mean ± standard error of the mean (SEM). Comparisons within groups were made by means of the Friedman nonparametric repeated measures test or the Mann-Whitney test where appropriate. The significance level was taken as a probability (two-sided) of < 0.05.

Results

IHP Study in Pigs

Operative Procedure. The duration of the operation ranged from 4 to 7 h (median 6 h), with a median blood loss of 500 ml (range 300–1500 ml). Stable perfusion was attained in all animals with no apparent leakage, as demonstrated by fluorescein dye injection. One pig died on the first postoperative day (necropsy revealed haemorrhagic ascites), but all other animals survived IHP without procedure-related complications. There was no significant renal, hematological, or cardiopulmonary toxicity.

Liver Function Tests and Chemistry. In all animals, including controls, significant initial elevations in ASAT, ALAT, lactate dehydrogenase (LDH), and alkaline phosphatase levels were observed (with peak values occurring on day 1 after

IHP), followed by gradual normalization within the first postoperative week. Total bilirubin, urea, γ-glutomyl transferase (γ-GT), and creatinine-values remained within the normal range (data not shown). There were no significant differences in peak values or kinetics between the three groups. Serum albumin levels decreased to a nadir of about 15 g/l at 1 h after IHP and returned to normal within the following 1–2 weeks. Platelet counts decreased slightly, but not significantly, during the first postoperative day and normalized within 3–7 days. There were no significant differences between groups.

TNFα Levels. TNFα levels in the perfusate increased to a median of 5.1×10^6 pg/ml (range 4.9×10^6 to 6.6×10^6) in both TNF-treated groups (< 5 pg/ml in the sham group) and remained virtually stable during the entire perfusion period. The cumulative leakage during IHP, as estimated from relative systemic TNFα levels, was less than 0.02%. However, at 1 min after declamping, systemic TNFα levels increased significantly in both TNF-treated groups, with peak levels ranging from 3.0×10^3 to 25×10^3 pg/ml, followed by rapid normalization over the next 6 h.

Histology. Compared with preperfusion histology, microscopic examination of HE-stained sections obtained directly after perfusion showed mild sinusoidal dilatation, as septal edema, and sporadic intraseptal polymorphonuclear neutrophil (PMN) infiltrations. At 4–6 weeks after perfusion, all microscopic sections revealed normal pig liver histology (on both HEE and electron microscopy) with the exception of sporadic polymorphonuclear neutrophil (PMN) infiltrates in the liver parenchyma. These findings were similar in all three groups.

Phase I Study

Operative Procedure. The median duration of the operation was 8 h (range 6–10 h). A stable perfusion was attained in all patients. Systemic leakage was demonstrated in only one patient during the IHP procedure. It resulted in discontinuing the IHP after 43 min (cumulative leakage 20%). Median blood loss was 5250 ml (range 4700–25 000 ml), including blood lost in the perfusion circuit. Three patients died during the perioperative period. One patient (no. 1) died from sepsis with multiple organ failure due to biliary tract necrosis that was a result of common hepatic artery thrombosis following iatrogenic hepatic artery injury. In the second patient (no. 2) there was an unacceptably large blood loss prior to drug administration, possibly caused by preoperative abuse of aspirin (unknown to the physician), which caused severe coagulopathy leading to exsanguination. The third patient (no. 3) (given 0.8 mg rhTNFα) was reoperated because of hypotension and shock about 25 min after a completely normal IHP procedure. Uncontrollable, diffuse intraperitoneal hemorrhage was demonstrated, probably caused by a coagulation disorder; it led to exsanguination. This adverse event was reported as prob-

Table 1. Toxicity (WHO grades) after isolated hepatic perfusion with tumor necrosis factor and melphalan

Parameter	Toxicity	
	Grade III	Grade IV
Blood pressure	0	1
Pulmonary function	0	2
Renal function	1	1
Hepatic function	2	3
White blood cell count	0	0
Platelets	0	0

WHO, World Health Organization

ably drug related rhTNFα, and the phase I study was discontinued. The remaining six patients (five men, one woman) survived the operation and were evaluable for tumor response.

Toxicity. Toxicity and adverse events were assessed and recorded according to the World Health Organization (WHO) grading system (WHO Adverse Event Coding Thesaurus) (Weber et al. 1993). Toxicity within the first 30 days after IHP is summarized in Table 1. Slight fever, hypotension, pulmonary hypertension, and sinus tachycardia were demonstrated in all patients and reported as drug-related. All patients demonstrated an anemia (nadir at day 3) and thrombocytopenia (nadir $69.2 \pm 14 \times 10^9/l$ at day 3), returning to normal 10 days after IHP. Furthermore, all patients demonstrated initial significantly elevated liver function tests, normalizing within the first 7–10 postoperative days (Fig. 1). Two patients had grade III and three grade IV hepatotoxicity. Some degree of pulmonary hypertension was demonstrated in almost all patients, with two patients developing adult respiratory distress syndrome (ARDS).

Survival. Among the six evaluable patients the survival time ranged from 6 to 26 months. The median survival time was 10.3 months (mean 13.3 months).

Tumor Response. The primary efficacy endpoints in the study were best tumor response observed [WHO response criteria: complete response (CR), partial response (PR), stable disease (SD), or progressive disease (PD)] and duration of the best response, calculated from the date the best response was observed until the date of progression. This best response was confirmed objectively in five patients by a true-cut biopsy and in the other patient by CT scan.

Among the six evaluable patients, five had partial responses and one had stable disease. In one patient (no. 1), a complete response was observed at autopsy 26 days after IHP. The duration of best response ranged from 17.5 to 32.5 weeks (median 18 weeks). The first sites of progression were the lung ($n=2$) and brain ($n=1$). In one other patient local recurrence of the primary tumor (rectal carcinoma) was observed. Two patients demonstrated local progression in the liver.

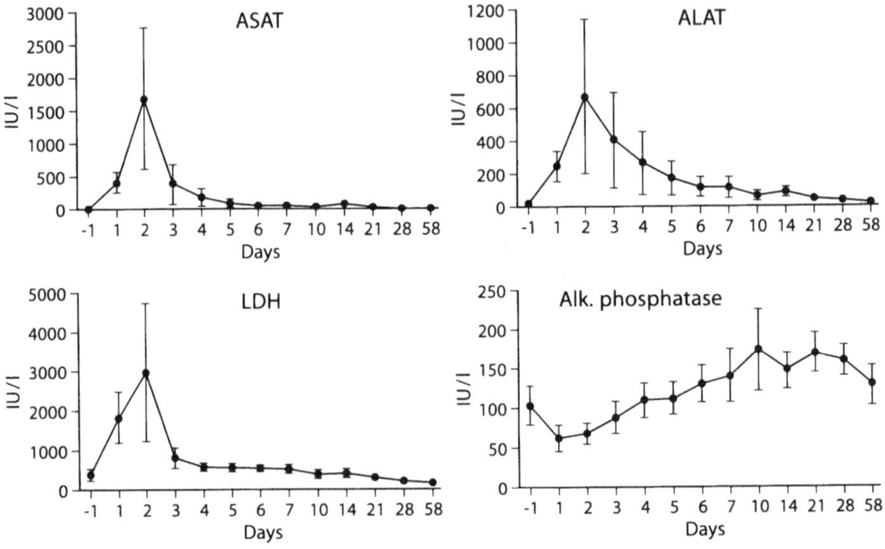

Fig. 1. Hepatic function tests after isolated hepatic perfusion with tumor necrosis factor and melphalan. *ASAT,* aspartate aminotransferase; *ALAT,* alanine aminotransferase; *LDH,* lactate dehydrogenase; *AIK. Fosfatase,* alkaline phosphatase

TNFα, Interleukin, and sTNFR Levels. In the perfusate the initial TNFα level of 1.8 ± 0.5 pg/ml increased rapidly to $6 \pm 2 \times 10^4$ pg/ml at 10 min, followed by a decrease to $2.8 \pm 0.9 \times 10^4$ pg/ml at the end of IHP. Interleukin 6 and 8 (IL-6, IL-8) levels increased significantly to $4 \pm 0.6 \times 10^3$ pg/ml, and $12 \pm 0.8 \times 10^3$ pg/ml respectively. Also sTNFR-p55 and sTNFR-p75 levels increased to 9.7 ± 0.8 ng/ml and 3.1 ± 0.8 ng/ml, respectively, at the end of IHP. Systemic levels of TNFα and both sTNFRs remained virtually unchanged during the IHP. After the wash-out, systemic TNFα levels increased rapidly to a peak value of 169 ± 38 pg/ml at 1 min and normalized within the next 2 h. IL-6 and IL-8 demonstrated a significant increase to peak levels of $9.8 \pm 0.8 \times 10^3$ pg/ml and $8.3 \pm 0.8 \times 10^3$ pg/ml, respectively at 60 min, thereafter decreasing to preoperative values. At 10 min after washout both sTNFR levels started to increase and remained significantly elevated during the following 2 weeks (de Vries et al. 1995a).

Acute-Phase Protein Levels. C-reactive protein (CRP) levels started to rise 9 h after washout and reached maximum levels (140.1 ± 19 mg/l) at the third postoperative day. Albumin decreased to 16.8 ± 0.1 g/l at 60 min, whereafter levels normalized. The "negative" acute-phase protein levels decreased to a nadir 30–60 min after washout, and levels normalized within the next 5 days. The other acute-phase proteins started to rise at 60 min after washout and were still elevated at day 10 (data not shown).

Coagulation and Fibrinolysis. In the perfusate, PAI levels were doubled at the end of IHP. In contrast, no significant changes occurred in TAT, PAP, and t-PA levels. After washout, systemic levels of all measured parameters increased significantly to peak values at 60–120 min, whereafter levels normalized (de Vries et al. 1995b).

Discussion

Several IHP methods were employed in the past (Skibba et al. 1983; Aigner 1988; De Brauw et al. 1988), that initially encountered technical difficulties resulting in incomplete vascular isolation and systemic leakage of drugs. In view of these findings, we modified the IHP technique in an attempt to minimize leakage. The first modification consisted of the development of a pump-aided, extracorporeal venovenous bypass shunt (VVB) as a second circuit during IHP. The VVB has the additional advantage of sufficiently shunting the blood from the lower body and intestines, resulting in better hemodynamic control during IHP. In fact, in the experimental animal study, no hemodynamic instability was observed during the experiments. During IHP, complete vascular isolation of the liver is essential to avoid systemic exposure to chemotherapeutic agents. We detected no significant leakage from the perfusion circuit to the systemic circulation in the pigs before adding rhTNF*α* to the perfusate, a finding confirmed in a quantitative analysis of systemic levels of TNF*α* during the vascular isolation period, which were about four orders of magnitude lower than the perfusate levels. Maximal cumulative leakage of rhTNF*α* from the perfusate was estimated to be less than 0.02%. In our clinical program vascular isolation was complete in all but one patient. In this patient the IHP had to be stopped after 43 min because of progressive systemic leakage (cumulative leakage 20%). Despite the leakage, with higher systemic TNF*α* levels during IHP this patient did not exhibit additional toxicity, demonstrated by clinical and biochemical parameters, compared to the other patients studied. In the eight patients with no leakage, systemic TNF*α* levels during the IHP did not change significantly, indicating that vascular isolation was complete. However, after the washout systemic TNF*α* levels rose - probably because of resorption of TNF*α* from the liver into the systemic circulation - and then normalized within the next 2 h. The second modification of the IHP technique involved the use of both hepatic artery and portal vein as inflow routes. Normal hepatic parenchyma receives most of its blood supply from branches of the portal vein and to a much lesser extent from the hepatic artery. In contrast, the blood supply of hepatic metastases has been ascribed to rely almost entirely on the hepatic artery, although small (< 5 mm) liver tumors and the outer rim of large hepatic metastases have been shown to be fed mainly by portal branches (Archer and Gray 1989, Strohmeyer et al. 1986). Most colorectal tumors drain via the portal vein suggesting that spreading tumor cells first proliferate in the portal system. Thus by using the hepatic artery and the portal vein drugs reach both established and newly formed (micro)metastases. Because most of the normal parenchyma is supplied primarily by the portal vein, it could be speculated that infusion via the portal vein might induce significant hepatotoxicity. In our animal study, however, we observed only mild, transient disturbances in liver enzymes and histology. Because these phenomena were also demonstrated in the control animals, the transient, mild hepatotoxicity observed probably has been caused by the IHP procedure itself; moreover addition of the drugs, in particular rhTNF*α*, does not lead to additional hepatotoxicity These findings are in agreement with those reported by others (Skibba et al. 1983). Our large animal study further demonstrates that hyperthermic isolated perfusion of the liver via the hepatic artery and portal vein is technically feasible and may be performed safely. The temporary exposure of normal porcine liver parenchyma to high-dose rhTNF*α* with and without melphalan followed by a washout procedure was well accepted.

After the successful and promising results of the preclinical pig study we started the phase I study of IHP with rhTNF*α* (0.4 mg in eight patients and 0.8 mg in one) and melphalan (1 mg/kg) in nine patients with unresectable colorectal metastases confined to the liver. In contrast to the pig program, protracted hepatic toxicity was encountered in five of nine patients. Furthermore, three patients died during the perioperative period. Only one of these deaths (no. 3) was possibly drug-related, after which the study was discontinued. Unfortunately, we were not able to evaluate coagulation and fibrinolysis in this patient by analyzing TAT, PAP, PAI, and t-PA levels. In the six evaluable patients, measurement of these parameters indicated significant activation of both coagulation and fibrinolysis.

The toxicity we encountered was higher than expected from the preclinical pig program. In two patients grade III hepatotoxicity and in three patients grade IV hepatotoxicity was shown. All patients developed some degree of pulmonary hypertension, with two patients developing ARDS. Kahky et al. (1990) demonstrated that intraportal administration of rhTNF*α* 100 μg/kg per day resulted in 100% mortality in rats. Histological examination demonstrated significant gastric and small intestinal mucosal injury, mild passive congestion of the liver, and severe pulmonary edema. Animals that had received rhTNF*α* systemically followed a relatively benign course with only mild pulmonary edema and no renal or gastrointestinal injury. Most hepatic Kupffer cells are situated in the (peri)portal area, and TNF*α* is known to induce production of various cytokines (including IL-1, IL-6, and TNF*α*) by macrophages (i.e., Kupffer cells). Hence this situation could be an explanation for the toxicity we encountered, as we performed IHP via the hepatic artery and the portal vein (Busam et al. 1990). Indeed high IL-6 and IL-8 levels were seen in our patients (de Vries et al. 1995b); and they were significantly higher than levels in the ILP setting (Swaak et al. 1993). Paradoxically, we could not demonstrate a significant correlation between peak levels of IL-6 or IL-8 and clinical parameters such as fever or hypotension. Furthermore, cytokine levels in two patients with ARDS were not different from those measured in the other patients. The investigated acute-phase proteins demonstrated the same course as in the ILP setting, with CRP reaching peak levels 48 h after IHP. There were no significant differences between patients.

A possible means of protection against TNFα is its soluble receptors. Depending on their concentration relative to TNFα, they may inhibit or augment (by acting as a slow-release buffer system) TNFα effects (Aderka et al. 1992). Levels of both receptors have been demonstrated to correlate with disease activity in various stages of cancer as well as sepsis (Aderka et al. 1991). Prolonged elevated levels of both sTNFRs were demonstrated in our patients, which is in accordance with these studies, indicating a protracted period of systemic inflammatory response syndrome, as seen in some of our patients (de Vries et al. 1995a).

In our phase I study, all patients who survived the IHP demonstrated a tumor response to the IHP. Furthermore, in the patient who died after multiple organ failure, described above, a complete response was demonstrated at autopsy. Unfortunately, the response was only temporary, with a range of 17.5–32.5 weeks. Eventually all patients relapsed locally or at a distant site, and all patients died of disease, with a median survival of 10.3 months (range 6–26 months).

Conclusion

Despite the promising experiences with our pig program, many problems were encountered during the phase I study. Contributing factors were the magnitude of the surgical procedure of IHP and the overall blood loss (median 5500 ml). By using both the hepatic artery and the portal vein in the IHP we encountered more toxicity than expected from the pig program, resulting in fatal coagulative disturbances in one patient who received the second rhTNFα dose. Furthermore, local control after one IHP with TNFα and melphalan is temporary. Taking into account the current aims and indications for IHP (i.e., to strive for hepatic tumor control in patients with distant metastases), it is clear that simplification and further optimization of the IHP technique is necessary to render it a smaller, preferably less invasive technique. One possibility that may be explored is the employment of multiple balloon catheters to achieve vascular isolation (Ku et al 1995).

References

Aderka D, Engelmann H, Hornik V, Skornick Y, Levo Y, Wallach D, Kusthai G (1991) Increased serum levels of soluble receptors for tumor necrosis factor in cancer patients. Cancer Res 51:5602–5607

Aderka D, Engelmann H, Maor Y, Brakebusch C, Wallach D (1992) Stabilization of the bioactivity of tumor necrosis factor by its soluble receptors. J Exp Med 175:323–329

Aigner KR (1988) Isolated liver perfusion: 5-year-results. Reg Cancer Treat 1:11–20

Archer SG, Gray BN (1989) Vascularization of small liver metastases. Br J Surg 76:545–548

Bordel Rinkes IHM, De Vries MR, Jonker AM, Swaak TJG, Hack CE, Nooijen PTGA, Wiggers T, Eggermont AMM (1997) Isolated hepatic perfusion in the pig with TNFα with and without melphalan. Br J Cancer (in press)
Busam KJ, Bauer TM, Bauer J, Gerok W, Decker B (1990) Interleukin-6 release by rat liver macrophages. J Hepatol 11:367–373
Carswell EA, Old JJ, Kassel RL, Green S, Fiore N, Williamson B (1975) An endotoxin induced serum factor that causes necrosis of tumours. Proc Natl Acad Sci USA 72:3666–3670
De Brauw LM, Van de Velde CJH, Tjaden LR, De Bruijn EA, Bell AVRJ, Hermans J, Zwaveling A (1988) In vivo isolated liver perfusion technique in a rat hepatic metastasis model: 5-fluorouracil concentrations in tumor tissue. J Surg Res 44:137–145
De Takats PG, Kerr DJ, Poole CJ, Warren HW, McArdle CS (1994) Hepatic arterial chemotherapy for metastatic colorectal carcinoma (review). Br J Cancer 69:372–378
Eggermont AMM, Schraffordt Koops H, Klausner JM et al (1996a) Isolated limb perfusion with tumor necrosis factor and melphalan for limb salvage in 186 patients with locally advanced soft tissue extremity sarcomas. The cumulative multicenter European experience. Ann Surg 224:756–765
De Vries MR, Borel Rinkes IHM, Buurman WA, Wiggers T, Van de Velde CJH, Eggermont AMM (1995a) Soluble TNFα receptor induction by isolated hepatic perfusion with TNFα and melphalan. Eur J Surg Res 27(S1):108
De Vries MR, Borel Rinkes IHM, Hack CE, Wiggers T, Van de Velde CJH, Kuppen PJK, Eggermont AMM (1995b) Isolated hepatic perfusion with TNFα and melphalan: local and systemic effects on secondary cytokine release, coagulation and fibrinolysis. Eur J Surg Res 27(S1):109
Eggermont AMM, Schraffordt Koops H, Lienard D, Kroon BBR, Van Geel AN, Hoekstra HJ, Lejeune FJ (1996b) Isolated limb perfusion with high-dose tumor necrosis factor α in combination with interferon γ and melphalan for nonresectable extremity soft tissue sarcomas: a multicenter trial. J Clin Oncol 14:2653–2665
Feinberg B, Kurzrock R, Talpaz M et al (1988) A phase I trial of intravenously administered recombinant tumor necrosis factor in patients with advanced cancer. J Clin Oncol 6:1328–1334
Genari L (1992) Liver metastases: a many-sided therapeutical problem. Hepatogastroenterology 39:5–9
Hack CE, Hart M, Strack van Schijndel A et al (1992) Interleukin-8 in sepsis: relation to shock and inflammatory mediators. Infect Immunol 60:2835–2842
Helle M, Boeije L, De Groot ER, De Vos A, Aarden LA (1991) Sensitive ELISA for interleukin-6. Detection of IL-6 in biological fluids: synovial fluids and sera. J Immunol Methods 138:42–56
Kahky MP, Daniel CO, Cruz AB, Gaskill HV (1990) Portal infusion of tumor necrosis factor increases mortality in rats. J Surg Res 49:138–145
Ku Y, Fukumoto T, Iwasaki T et al (1995) Clinical pilot study with high-dose intraarterial chemotherapy with direct hemoperfusion under hepatic venous isolation in patients with advanced hepatocellular carcinoma. Surgery 117:510–519
Leeuwenberg JFM, Jeunhomme TMAA, Buurman WA (1994) Slow release of soluble TNF receptors by monocytes in vitro. J Immunol 152:4036–4043
Lienard D, Ewalenko P, Delmotte JJ, Renard N, Lejeune FJ (1992) High-dose recombinant tumor necrosis factor alpha in combination with interferon gamma and melphalan in isolated perfusion of the limbs for melanoma and sarcoma. J Clin Oncol 10:50–62
Manusama ER, Nooijen PTGA, Stavast J, Durante NMC, Marquet RL, Eggermont AMM (1996) Synergistic antitumor effect of recombinant human tumor necrosis factor α with melphalan in isolated limb perfusion in the rat. Br J Surg 83:551–555
Marinelli A, Dijkstra FR, Van Dierendonck JH, Kuppen PJK, Cornelisse CJ, Van de Velde CJH (1991) Effectiveness of isolated liver perfusion with mitomycin C in the treatment of liver tumor of rat colorectal cancer. Br J Cancer 64:74–78
Que FG, Nagorney DM (1994) Resection of 'recurrent' colorectal metastases to the liver. Br J Surg 81:255–258

Renard N, Lienard D, Lespagnard L, Eggermont AMM, Heimann R, Lejeune FJ (1994) Early endothelium activation and polymorphonuclear cell invasion precede specific necrosis of human melanoma and sarcoma treated by intravascular high-dose tumor necrosis factor alpha (TNFα) Int J Cancer 57:656–663

Skibba JL, Almagro UA, Condon RE, Petroff RJ Jr (1983) A technique for isolated perfusion of the canine liver with survival. J Surg Res 34:123–132

Spriggs DR, Sherman ML, Micjie H et al (1988) Recombinant human tumor necrosis factor administered as a 24-hour intravenous infusion. A phase I and pharmacological study. J Natl Cancer Inst 80:1039–1044

Strohmeyer T, Haugeberg G, Lierse W (1986) Vaskularisation von Lebermetastasen: eine korrosionsanatomische Studie. Acta Anat (Basel) 126:172–176

Swaak AJG, Lienard D, Schrafforgt Koops H, Lejeune FJ, Eggermont AMM (1993) Effects of recombinant tumour necrosis factor (rTNFa) in cancer. Observations on the acute phase protein reaction and immunoglobulin synthesis after high dose rTNFa administration in isolated limb perfusions in cancer patients. Eur J Clin Invest 23:812–818

Vreugdenhil G, Lowenberg B, Van Eijk HG, Swaak AJ (1992) Tumor necrosis factor alpha is associated with disease activity and the degree of anemia in patients with rheumatoid arthritis. Eur J Clin Invest 22:488–493

Wagner JS, Adson MA, Van Heerden JA, Adson MH, Ilstrup DM (1984) The natural history of hepatic metastases from colorectal origin. A comparison with resective treatment. Ann Surg 199:502–508

Weber J, Yang JC, Topalian SL et al (1993) Phase I trial of subcutaneous interleukin-6 in patients with advanced malignancies. J Clin Oncol 11:499–506

Isolated Hepatic Perfusion with Extracorporeal Oxygenation Using Hyperthermia TNFα and Melphalan: Swedish Experience*

L. Hafström[1] and P. Naredi[2]

[1] Department of Surgery, University Hospital, S-901 85 Umeå, Sweden
[2] Department Surgery, Sahlgrenska University Hospital, S-41345 Gothenburg, Sweden

Abstract

A phase I trial was performed to determine the toxicity and efficacy of isolated hepatic perfusion with tumour necrosis factorα (TNF) and melphalan (Alkeran) under mild hyperthermic conditions. Eleven patients with unresectable metastatic malignancies in the liver (malignant melanoma, leiomyosarcoma, colorectal cancer) underwent the procedure. Compared to our earlier experience with melphalan and *cis*-platinum under hyperthermic conditions (41.7 °C), this phase I study with TNF 30–200 μg and melphalan 0.5 mg/kg body weight under 39 °C hyperthermia neither improved the response rate nor decreased the serious adverse effects. Two patients died within the first postoperative month owing to coagulopathy or multiple organ failure. Five patients were reoperated owing to postoperative bleeding. Three of six patients with liver metastases from malignant melanoma or leiomyosarcoma and none of five patients with liver metastases from colorectal cancer showed a partial response.

Historical Background

As early as 1960 two papers described the technique for isolated chemotherapy perfusion of the liver using an extracorporeal circuit (Aust and Ausman 1960; Healey 1960). Ausman and Aust presented their studies at the Surgical Forum in the United States on leakage during hepatic perfusion in dogs, and in 1961 Ausman reported his findings of perfusion in five patients. Stehlin, one of the pioneers in isolated limb perfusion collaborated with Healey et al. (1961) when they studied the hepatic tolerance of thiotepa in dogs using an isolation technique.

* Supported by grants from the Swedish Medical Research Foundation (grant K97-17X-07184-13A) and the Swedish Cancer Society (grant 1081-B96-11XAB). TNFα was kindly supplied by Hans Kierulff-Nielsen, Interferon Research Institute, Hjörring, Denmark.

Recent Results in Cancer Research, Vol. 147

In 1983 Aigner et al. presented the first clinical results of isolated hepatic perfusion with 5-fluorouracil on two patients suffering liver metastases from colorectal cancer. In this study a temperature of 38.1 °C for 1 h was used. They found that the metastases showed central necrosis and that there were no side effects or complications within 6 months after the perfusion. Later Aigner et al. (1988) reported a 67% remission rate of colorectal liver metastases treated with isolated hepatic perfusion with mitomycin C and 5-fluorouracil. In this study more regional infusion therapy was administered after the perfusion.

Theoretical Background

The advantage of regional isolation perfusion therapy versus systemic therapy is well established. By administrating the drug to an isolated organ (liver) with cancer, a higher regional drug concentration can be achieved, as the drug is mixed and diluted in a smaller volume (i.e., the blood volume of the organ and the extracorporeal perfusion system). If there is complete isolation of the organ with no leakage and if the organ is cleared of the drug before the isolation is released and normal flow reestablished, systemic toxic effects can be avoided.

Furthermore, there is an additive or synergistic effect between certain chemotherapeutic drugs and increased temperature. The regional isolation perfusion technique makes it possible to apply hyperthermia during the perfusion.

The disadvantages of the technique are the short duration of drug exposure, local toxicity, and the complicated method required for complete isolation. The possibilities for repeated perfusions are also limited.

Practical Background

A vast experience with hyperthermic melphalan limb perfusion for melanomas has been of importance when establishing isolated hepatic perfusion. Approximately 80% complete and partial remissions of the tumour can be achieved with isolated limb perfusion for melanoma. (Hafström and Mattsson 1993). As the technique for isolating the liver for perfusion is similar to that for isolating the liver for transplantation, experience in orthotopic liver transplantation is advantageous.

In 1985 the first isolated hepatic perfusion with melphalan was performed on a patient with malignant melanoma secondary to an ocular melanoma. The patient experienced significant tumour reduction and survived more than four years after the perfusion.

The first series of isolated hepatic perfusions included 29 patients on whom 30 perfusions with melphalan (0.5 mg/kg) were performed (Hafström et al. 1994 a, b). The maximum temperature in the perfusion circuit was

41.7 °C, and the flow was about 1000 ml/min. Twenty patients were also given cis-platinum in an escalating dose from 0.2 to 0.7 mg. This first series showed that perfusion of the liver and decompression of the lower caval vein and the portal vein with an internal Perfufix caval shunt was feasible. Partial tumour remission was observed in 20% of the patients in this study, although mortality and morbidity were significant in patients with a liver tumour volume of more than 50%. Four patients died within 30 days due to multiorgan failure (Hafström et al. 1994a).

Based on the experience with tumour necrosis factor α (TNF) in isolated limb perfusions of melanoma lesions by Lejeune and others (Lienard et al. 1992) TNF hepatic perfusions were started in 1992. The aim of the study was to determine if it was feasible to give TNF in an isolated hepatic perfusion system with melphalan (Alkeran) and hyperthermia. Eleven patients have so far been treated with the protocol.

Technique for Isolated Hepatic Perfusion with TNF and Melphalan

Preoperative evaluation includes standard liver function tests. A computed tomographic (CT) scan [or magnetic resonance imaging (MRI) scan] is mandatory to evaluate tumour volume in the liver and to exclude major extrahepatic growth. A CT (or MRI) scan of the brain is always performed in patients with malignant melanoma. Liver angiography to map the vascular anatomy of the liver is considered valuable.

The patients were given Human Leukocyte Interferon (Interferon Research Institute, Hjörring, Denmark) 3×10^6 units daily 2 days before operation to up-regulate TNF receptors.

A bilateral subcostal incision is made under general anaesthesia. Initially the intra- and extrahepatic tumour volumes are evaluated. If the patient is then considered suitable for hyperthermic hepatic perfusion, the gastroduodenal artery, proper hepatic artery, and portal vein are isolated (Fig. 1). The infrahepatic caval vein is isolated above the renal veins and the suprahepatic caval vein between the diaphragm and the pericardium. Tributaries from behind and from the diaphragm are occluded separately, as are the veins from the right suprarenal gland. Wire-reinforced catheters are inserted via the saphenous vein to the iliac vein, in the axillary vein, in the testicular vein (or ovarian vein) to the retrohepatic portion of the caval vein, via the inferior mesenteric vein to the portal vein, via the gastroduodenal artery to the proper hepatic artery, and in the portal vein.

An external shunt from the iliac vein and from the portal vein through a centrifugal pump to the axillary vein is applied (Fig. 1). The perfusion system is primed with Ringer's solution. After that the perfusion circuit from the hepatic caval vein to the portal vein and the proper hepatic artery is applied. In the perfusion circuit there is a roller pump, an oxygenator (Minimax Hollowfiber oxygenator), tubing (Carmeda Bioactive Surface Catheters, or CBAS), and a heater. The infrahepatic caval vein is occluded with a linen

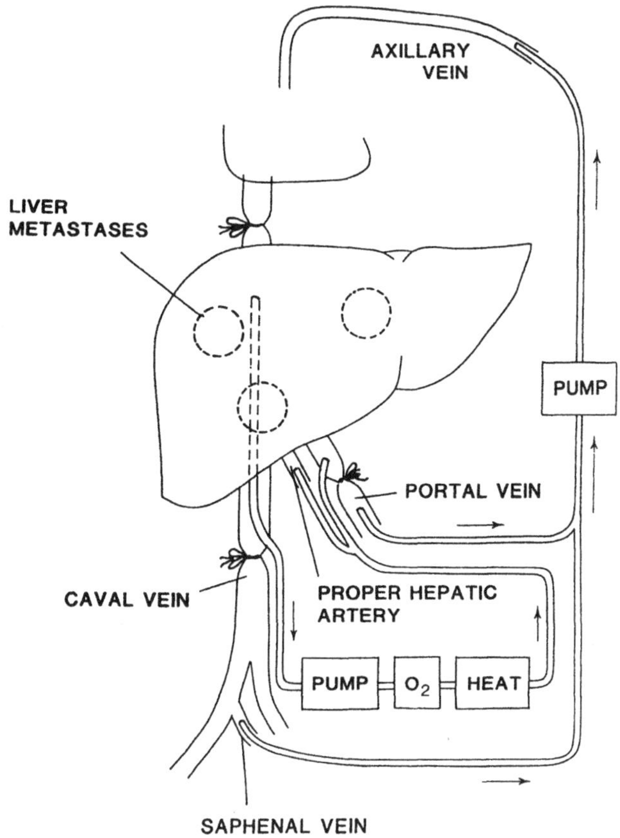

Fig. 1. Technique for isolated hepatic perfusion using an external shunt and a perfusion circuit

band, and the suprahepatic caval vein and portal vein proximal to the inflow catheter are occluded with vascular clamps.

A flow of 1000–1500 ml/min is established in the perfusion circuit. The temperature is initially maintained at 37 °C and is continuously measured by thermistor probes placed in the inflow catheters, the liver parenchyma, and the liver tumours. It is recorded with the MedicView computerised system.

When steady state is established in the perfusion circuit and there is no sign of leakage, TNFα (Interferon Research Institute) is administered into the perfusion circuit. The first four patients received TNF 0.5 µg/kg, the following four patients 100 µg, and the last three 200 µg. After 30 min of perfusion with TNF, the temperature in the inflow is increased to 41 °C and then to 39 °C in the liver parenchyma; melphalan 0.5 mg/kg is then administered. The perfusion is continued for another 60 min, whereafter the perfusion is discontinued and the liver is irrigated with 1000 ml low-molecular-weight dextran (Rheomacrodex). The shunts and perfusion circuit are disconnected and the procedure is concluded.

The mesenteric vein, testicular vein, and saphenous vein are ligated, as is the gastroduodenal artery. The incisions in the axillary vein and the portal vein are sutured. Postoperatively, the patients are cared for at the intensive care unit (ICU) for a median of 4 days.

Results

Eleven patients with unresectable liver tumours have been treated. Two patients had metastases from ocular malignant melanoma, four had leiomyosarcomas, and five had liver metastases from colorectal cancer. These patients had no evidence of macroscopic extrahepatic tumour growth. The median duration of surgery was 6 h (range 4.5–6.5 h), and the median blood loss was 5 l (range 1–42 l). Six patients were reoperated. One patient had bile leakage due to necrotic metastases, and five patients were reoperated because of postoperative bleeding within 24 h. At the time of reoperation, generally no major bleeding sites were found.

An elevation in liver transaminases was seen after 3–5 days [aspartate aminotransferase (AST) 23 ± 10 µkat/ml, alanine aminotransferase (ALT) 9 ± 3 µkat/ml] followed by an elevation in serum bilirubin (85 ± 43 µmol/l) a few days later. One patient in whom more than 75% of the liver volume was occupied with metastases of leiomyosarcoma had hepatorenal syndrome. She recovered after 27 days at the ICU. One patient developed a fatal coagulopathy during surgery and succumbed within the first postoperative 24 h. One patient succumbed due to multiple organ failure.

Tumour Effect and Survival

Tumour remission was assessed by CT scan or MRI every 2 months using UICC criteria. Clinical progression or death before the first evaluation was considered progressive disease. Three patients had a partial response, with times to progression of 5, 7, and 8 months, respectively. Six patients had stable disease for 2–10 months. Two patients succumbed within the first postoperative month owing to treatment complications. One of two patients with malignant melanoma, two of four with leiomyosarcoma, and none of five with a colorectal primary cancer showed a response (Table 1).

Measurement of TNF*α*

Tumor necrosis factor was measured before administration and during the perfusion. Using the enzyme-linked immunosorbent assay (ELISA; Amersham) and a bioassay (L929 cells with actinomycin D 1 µg/ml added) the elevated TNF concentrations in the perfusate were measured throughout the perfusion without signs of significant leakage from the perfusion circuit.

Table 1. Tumour response and survival after isolated hepatic perfusion with TNF and melphalan

Patient	Tumour type	TNF dose (μg)	Tumour response	Survival (months)
1	Leiomyosarcoma	40	PR	18
2	Melanoma	40	PR	8
3	Melanoma	30	SD	34+
4	Colorectal	50	SD	7
5	Leiomyosarcoma	100	SD	10
6	Leiomyosarcoma	100	PR	19
7	Leiomyosarcoma	100	SD	21+
8	Colorectal	100	PD	0
9	Colorectal	200	SD	15+
10	Golorectal	200	PD	0
11	Golorectal	200	SD	8+

PR, partial response; *SD*, stable disease; *PD*, progressive disease; +, patient is alive

Peak concentrations in the perfusate measured with ELISA varied considerably (1–75% of the administered TNF dose) in the various patients. TNF concentrations measured by the bioassay corresponded to the administered doses. The disadvantage of the bioassay is that it is unreliable after melphalan is added to the perfusate. To further clarify if there was significant leakage from the perfusion circuit or if there was a considerable first-passage uptake of TNF in the liver, an in vitro experiment resembling a perfusion but without a patient was carried out. The CBAS system was used. The perfusate consisted of 100 ml plasma, 300 ml erythrocytes, and 300 ml Ringer's solution. The perfusate (pH 6.8) was oxygenated (pO_2 10–20 kPa) and heated to 37 °C. The test was performed with 1500 units of heparin (control) or without heparin. TNF was added in increasing doses from 50 μg up to 1500 μg. Samples were obtained 1 and 5 min after adding TNF. TNF concentrations were measured by ELISA and bioassay. The results (Table 2) show that the TNF concentrations measured by ELISA are significantly underestimated, especially in doses under 500 μg. This finding is in accordance with clinical data on TNF concentrations in liver perfusate reported by our group (Hafström et al. 1994b) and others (Jaskowiak et al. 1996) where 8% and 21%, respectively, of the administered dose in the perfusate was detected by ELISA.

Conclusion

It is feasible to perform isolated hepatic perfusion with TNF and melphalan in a hyperthermic oxygenated system. Compared to earlier experience with melphalan and *cis*-platinum under hyperthermic conditions, using TNF in doses up to 200 μg and melphalan 0.5 mg/kg under 39 °C hyperthermia neither improved the final response rate nor decreased the serious adverse ef-

Table 2. Measured TNF doses with ELISA and bioassay in vitro in the CBAS perfusion circuit

TNF added (μg)	L929/no heparin (μg)	ELISA/no heparin (μg)	ELISA/heparin (μg)
0		0	0
50	58	0	0
100	143	16	28
200	228	60	30
500	488	147	112
1500	1500	495	225

CBAS, Carmeda Bioactive Surface Catheters; *TNF*, tumour necrosis factor; *L929*, bioassay using L929 cells with actinomycin D 1 μg/ml, *ELISA*, enzyme-linked immunosorbent assay (Amersham kit); *no heparin*, CBAS system without added heparin; *heparin*, CBAS system with 1500 units of heparin added the perfusate

fects. Three of six patients with liver metastases from malignant melanoma or leiomyosarcoma and none of the five patients with liver metastases from colorectal cancer showed a partial response.

References

Aigner KR, Walther H, Tonn J, Wenzl A, Hechtel R, Merker G, Schwemmle K (1983) First experimental and clinical results of isolated hepatic perfusion with cytotoxics in metastases from colorectal primary. Recent Results Cancer Res 86:99–102

Aigner KR, Walther H, Link KH (1988) Isolated liver perfusion with MMC/5-Fu: surgical technique, pharmacokinetics, clinical results. Contrib Oncol 29:229–246

Ausman RK (1961) Development of a technic for isolated perfusion of the liver. NY State J Med 61:3993–3997

Ausman RK, Aust JB (1960) Isolated perfusion of the liver with HN_2. Surg Forum 10:77

Aust JB, Ausman RK (1960) The technique of liver perfusion. Cancer Chemother Rep 10:23–33

Hafström L, Mattson J (1993) Regional chemotherapy for malignant melanoma. Cancer Treat Rev 19:17–28

Hafström L, Holmberg SB, Naredi P, Lindnér PG, Bengtsson A, Tidebrant G, Scherstén T (1994a) Isolated hyperthermic liver perfusion with chemotherapy for liver malignancy. Surg Oncol 3:103–108

Hafström L, Holmberg SB, Lindnér PL, Naredi P, Asztely M, Bengtsson A, Nielsen HK, Scherstén T (1994b) Isolated regional liver perfusion with tumour necrosis factor-alpha followed by hyperthermic melphalan perfusion. Reg Cancer Treat 7:172–176

Healey JE (1960) The technique of liver perfusion. Cancer Chemother Rep 10:24

Healey JE, Smith JL, Clark RL, Stehlin JS, White EG (1961) Hepatic tissue tolerance to thio-TEPA administered by the isolation-perfusion technique. J Surg Res 1:111–116

Jaskowiak NT, Alexander HR, Bartlett DL, Turner EM, Tsigos C, Papanicolaou D, Chrousos GP, Fraker DL (1996) Secondary cytokine production and endocrine effects after high dose intravascular TNF. In: Fraker DL, Jacobsen SE (eds) TNF and related cytokines: clinical utility and biology of action. Cambridge Symposia, Hilton Head Island, South Carolina, p 8

Lienard D, Lejeune FJ, Ewalenko P (1992) In transit metastases of malignant melanoma treated by high dose rTNF-alpha in combination with interferon-gamma and melphalan in isolation perfusion. World J Surg 16:234–240

V. Radiological Control of Tumor Response

Role of Ultrasonography for Monitoring Tumor Necrosis After Chemotherapy

M. Gross[1] and W. G. Zoller[2]

[1] Medizinische Poliklinik, Klinikum Innenstadt, Ludwig-Maximilians-Universität München, Pettenkoferstraße 8a, D-80336 München, Germany
[2] Klinik für Allgemeine Innere Medizin, Katharinenhospital, Kriegsbergstraße 60, D-70174 Stuttgart, Germany

Abstract

Ultrasonography for monitoring the response of malignant liver lesions to regional therapy offers several advantages. The instrument is easy to transport and can be used in intensive care units, so it is the procedure of choice within the first few days after invasive techniques, such as isolated liver perfusion, to demonstrate tumor response. Changes in size or in the sonomorphological pattern of liver lesions early after therapy indicate a therapeutic response. There are no data available on the sensitivity of ultrasonography for differentiating the necrotic and viable parts of the tumor. If information on the extent of tumor necrosis is crucial for decisions on further treatment of a patient, ultrasonography should be complemented with other techniques, such as fine-needle puncture or imaging techniques such as computed tomography, nuclear magnetic resonance, and single photon emission computed tomography. The contribution of more recent developments in ultrasonography, such as color Doppler analysis of intratumoral blood flow or three-dimensional ultrasonography, for monitoring tumor necrosis remains to be evaluated.

Introduction

The number of alternative treatment regimens for primary or metastastic liver cancer has increased, offering usually more than one approach in a given patient. Evaluation of the efficacy of the various regimens is essential to offer the best approach to the patient.

The best criteria for the success of a therapeutic regimen are well-defined clinical endpoints, such as the 5-year survival rate or the mean duration of disease-free survival, but evaluation of treatment efficacy based on these criteria takes a long time. In addition, the need for early changes of treatment for nonresponders requires criteria that can be evaluated soon after the initiation of therapy.

Recent Results in Cancer Research, Vol. 147

When the efficacy of a treatment regimen for malignant liver lesions is to be evaluated, sequential ultrasonographic examinations of the patients may be a valuable tool. As a widely used noninvasive method, it can be repeated often and can even be used in the setting of an intensive care unit without the need to move the patient to other departments.

Sonographic Parameters of Liver Lesions with Prognostic Relevance

The basic sonomorphological characteristics of treatment-induced tumor regression of malignant liver lesions was reported more than 20 years ago (Gilby and Taylor 1975). After successful chemotherapy of a patient with liver metastases from a testicular teratoma, the initially hypoechoic, homogeneous lesion became hyperechoic and heterogeneous and then decreased in size. Finally, the lesion was no longer visible, and the patient was free of disease. In contrast, another patient with a liver metastasis from a small-cell lung cancer showed no changes in the sonomorphological pattern of the liver lesion during chemotherapy. The metastasis kept growing, and the patient died from progressive disease.

More than 20 years later these principles are still correct. Changes of the sonomorphological features of liver lesions and a decrease in size after the onset of chemotherapy indicate a therapeutic response to the treatment regimen (Fig.1). An unchanged sonographic pattern and an increase in size indicate progressive disease.

These statements are not as self-evident as they seem. For example, with esophageal cancer tumor regression due to radiochemotherapy is better predicted by clinical information, such as relief of dysphagia, or by bulk reduction seen by computed tomography (CT) or endoscopy. Endoscopic ultrasonography shows no decrease in tumor size after therapy because of T3 overstaging caused by the inflammatory reaction, which cannot be differentiated from viable tumor (Hordijk et al. 1993).

Several sonographic features of liver lesions can be determined by serial ultrasonography during therapy: number and size (diameter or surface) of the lesions, size of the largest lesion, echogenicity, homogeneity or the cluster type of lesions. The prognostic value of these variables was evaluated in various studies. A group of 42 patients with liver metastases (mainly from cancer of breast or lung or from colorectal cancer) were studied during a total of 123 cycles of chemotherapy (Bleiberg et al. 1989). The main criterion of a partial response was found to be regression of the metastatic surface (sum of the products of the largest perpendicular diameter of two lesions) by 50% or more. Several other studies also found that the decrease in size is the sonographic parameter with the highest prognostic value.

There is one major disadvantage to using tumor reduction as an indicator of tumor response to therapy. Because the reduction takes some time, it is not a suitable parameter to evaluate the immediate response to such procedures as chemoembolisation or regional liver perfusion or other types of re-

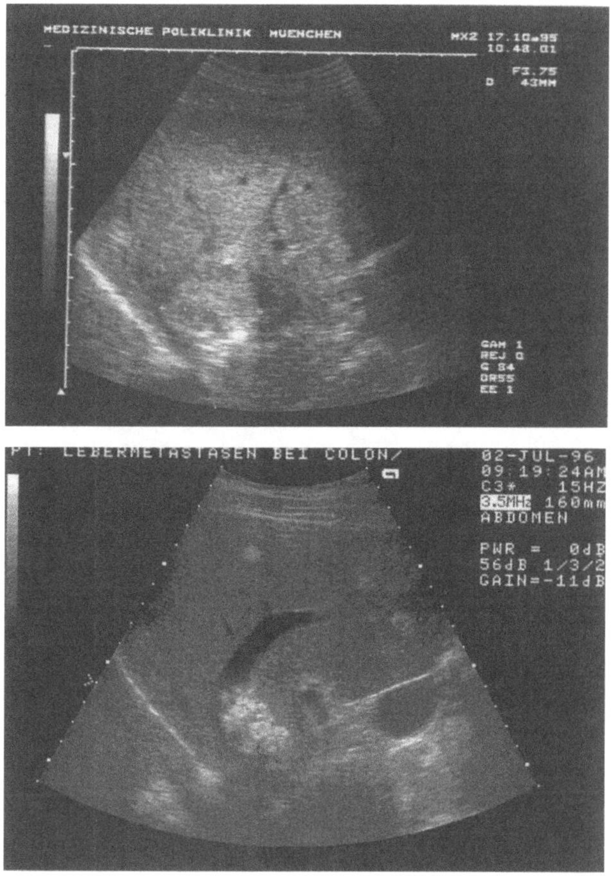

a

b

Fig. 1. a Sonography of a 54-year-old patient with liver metastases of a colorectal cancer prior to therapy. Multiple solid liver lesions can be seen, mainly isoechoic or hyperechoic. Some of the lesions are heterogeneous. **b** Sonography of the same patient 8 months after surgical resection of the colorectal cancer and regional chemotherapy of the liver using an intraarterial port system. The liver lesions strongly increased in echogenicity and decreased in size

gional therapy. To detect an early response under these therapeutic regimens, changes in the sonographic patterns are more helpful.

In most cases liver metastases or hepatocellular carcinoma are initially hypoechoic or isoechoic. In one study these characteristic was found in 80% of patients with liver metastases from various primary tumors (Görg et al. 1990): 80% of the metastases exhibited the typical halo sign, a hypoechoic rim surrounding the lesion. After successful therapy, hypoechoic lesions usually become hyperechoic or heterogeneous, and homogenously hyperechoic lesions become heterogeneous (Figs. 1, 2). This change is also the typical response of hepatocellular carcinoma to percutaneous ethanol injection (Shiina et al. 1987). Shiina et al. reported 18 patients with single lesions and 12 patients with multiple lesions. Before treatment most of the lesions were

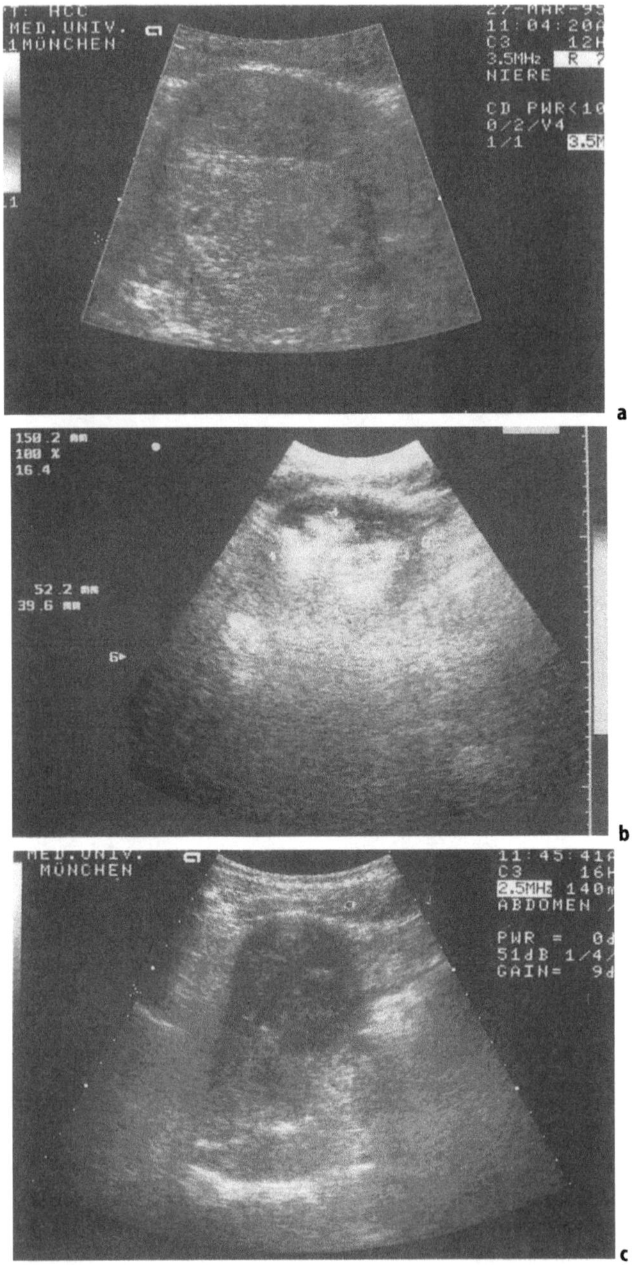

Fig. 2. a Sonography of the left liver lobe of a 71-year-old patient with a hepatocellular carcinoma prior to therapy. Note the inhomogeneous lesion with the halo sign. **b** Sonography of the same patient 2 days after chemoembolization of the lesion. The lesion is now hyperechoic without a significant change in size compared to the initial finding. **c** Sonography of the same patient 5 weeks after chemoembolization. The echogenicity became hypoechoic again. The heterogeneity is presumably due to necrotic portions of the tumor

hypoechoic, whereas after ethanol injection, they mainly became hyperechoic or heterogeneous.

Correlation Between Ultrasonography and Histology When Predicting Tumor Response

Immediate or early changes of the sonomorphological features are likely to represent tumor necrosis after local therapy of liver lesions. However, after therapy with ethanol injection or chemoembolisation it cannot be excluded that the changes represent only the presence of drugs delivered to the tumor. For example, after ethanol injection the immediate increase in echogenicity may be caused by destruction of regular liver tissue due to the relatively large volume of fluid injected into the lesion. If physiological saline is injected instead of ethanol, a similar increase in echogenicity is observed, indicating that early changes in echogenicity do not automatically indicate tumor necrosis. Therefore studies that compare changes in ultrasonography with changes in histology are crucial.

There is limited information in the literature on the value of ultrasonography for monitoring tumor necrosis during systemic chemotherapy and almost no data on the use of local chemotherapy. No studies have appeared on ultrasonography in patients with isolated liver perfusion.

One of the few studies correlating the changes seen by ultrasonography with those observed histologically was performed in 19 patients with liver metastases of colorectal cancers and 5 patients with hepatocellular carcinoma (Krakamp et al. 1990) These patients were treated by repeated regional intraarterial chemotherapy with 5-fluorouracil (5FU) and 1,3-bis-(2-chloroethyl)-I-nitrosourea (BCNU) every 2 weeks. Ultrasound-guided fine-needle puncture samples were obtained every 6 weeks, and the patients were studied repeatedly by ultrasonography of the liver.

Of the 19 patients with metastatic liver disease, 13 histologically showed regression initially. There was no change in the sonomorphological patterns of the liver lesions in 11 of these 13 patients, and sonographic evidence for a tumor response was found in only 2 patients. Six patients with initial regression confirmed by fine-needle puncture suffered subsequent histological progression. At that time, evidence for tumor progression was also demonstrated by ultrasonography in five of these six patients; no change was observed in the sixth patient.

No histological evidence for tumor regression was ever seen in six patients, despite chemotherapy. The sonographic findings in these patients were highly heterogeneous (no change in three patients, progression in two patients, regression in one patient).

The correlation was no better in patients with hepatocellular carcinoma. Histologically, tumor progression was seen in four of the five patients. Again, the sonographic findings in these patients were heterogeneous: progression in two patients and regression in the other two. At the time of the first histological evidence of tumor progression (n=5), the sonographic findings suggested tumor progression in only two patients, regression in two patients, and no change in one patient.

Obviously, the ultrasonographic findings did not correlate highly with the histological changes. If progression was seen by ultrasonography, the metastasis was indeed growing. In contrast, if no change was seen, the lesion histologically showed anything from regression to progression. If regression was suspected by ultrasonography, some of the lesions showed histological evidence of tumor progression. Only complete disappearance of the lesion or an increase in size clearly indicated tumor regression or progression, respectively.

Is the histological response indeed the gold standard with which ultrasonography can be compared? The survival time of the patients supports this hypothesis. The patients with histological evidence of tumor regression showed a mean survival of 12.0 ± 9.2 months (tumor regression first seen at a mean interval of 3.0 ± 0.7 months after initiation of therapy). In contrast, patients with histological evidence of tumor progression lived for a mean of only 4.5 ± 2.2 months after beginning therapy.

Recent Developments in Ultrasonography

The studies discussed before were performed using conventional ultrasound technology. Are there new ultrasonographic techniques that may help in future to predict tumor response?

One possibility is the combination of ultrasonography with color Doppler analysis. Changes of the Doppler signal in the arteries feeding the tumor are indicative of a tumor response, especially an increase in resistive index, as shown during preoperative chemotherapy for osteosarcoma (van der Woude et al. 1995). In that study, not only the velocity waveform in the arteries feeding the limb were analyzed but also the spectral waveform of blood vessels within the tumor. Persistent intratumoral flow and high-frequency Doppler shifts suggest a poor response, but these findings cannot easily be applied to liver lesions. The feeding artery most often cannot be visualized in the case of intrahepatic lesions, which is a prerequisite for Doppler analysis. Several studies on intratumoral blood flow of liver tumors measured by color Doppler analysis have been reported, but this technique does not seem to be reliable enough to be used for clinical studies (Ohnishi and Nomura 1989; Tanaka et al. 1990, 1992).

Another more recent development is three-dimensional (3D) ultrasonography. This technique results in better visualization of the intrahepatic lesions and adjacent structures, such as vessels and the diaphragm. The method employed by our group consists of a regular ultrasound machine (Acuson) with a curved array transducer. On top of the transducer is a small marker whose position in the room is registered by a sensor located below the patient. During the recording time of a few seconds, the transducer is slowly moved by hand across the lesion. At the same time, the computer is recording the individual ultrasound pictures (up to 25 pictures per second). This data set is passed on to a computer system that calculates 3D reconstruction. These reconstruction can be presented in several ways similar to the 3D reconstruction known from CT or MRI.

With 3D ultrasonography it is possible to calculate the exact volume of the lesion and thus to detect a decrease in size early after chemotherapy (Liess et al. 1994). It remains to be evaluated if 3D ultrasonography increases the diagnostic information gained from sonographic investigation of a patient in terms of the differential diagnosis of focal liver masses and the discrimination of necrotic versus viable parts of a liver tumor during therapy.

References

Bleiberg H, Gerard B, Peetrons PH, Dodion P (1989) Measurements of response to chemotherapy using ultrasound in metastatic liver involvement. Eur J Cancer Clin Oncol 25:857–859

Gilby ED, Taylor KJW (1975) Ultrasound monitoring of hepatic metastases during chemotherapy. BM J 1:371–373

Görg C, Schwerk WB, Wolf M, Havemann K (1990) Prognostic value of response to chemotherapy using ultrasound in lung cancer with metastatic liver involvement. Bildgebung 57:70–73

Hordijk ML, Kok TC, Wilson JHP, Mulder AH (1993) Assessment of response of esophageal carcinoma to induction chemotherapy. Endoscopy 25:592–596

Krakamp B, Schmitz R, Knöpfle G, Leidig P (1990) Primäre und metastatische Lebertumore – Beurteilung der Tumorregression bzw. -response unter regionaler Zytostase durch Sonographie und Feinnadelpunktionshistologie. Leber Magen Darm 3:138–144

Liess H, Roth C, Umgelter A, Zoller WG (1994) Improvements in volumetric quantification of circumscribed hepatic lesions by three dimensional sonography. Z Gastroenterol 32:488–492

Ohnishi K, Nomura F (1989) Ultrasonic Doppler studies of hepatocellular carcinoma and comparison with other hepatic focal lesions. Gastroenterology 97:1489–1497

Shiina 5, Yasuda J, Muto H, Tagawa K, Unuma T, Ibukuro K, Inoue Y, Takanashi R (1987) Percutaneous ethanol injection in the treatment of liver neoplasms. AJR Am J Roentgenol 149:949–952

Tanaka S, Kitamura T, Fujita M, Nakanishi K, Okuda S (1990) Color Doppler flow imaging of liver tumors. AJR Am J Roentgenol 154:509–514

Tanaka S, Kitamura T, Fujita M, Kasugai H, Inoue A, Ishiguro S (1992) Small hepatocellular carcinoma: differentiation from adenomatous hyperplastic nodule with color Doppler flow imaging. Radiology 182:161–165

Van der Woude H-J, Bloem JL, van Oostayen JA, Nooy MA, Taminiau AHM, Hermans J, Reynierse M, Hogendoorn PCW (1995) Treatment of high-grade bone sarcomas with neoadjuvant chemotherapy: the utility of sequential color Doppler sonography in predicting histopathological response. AJR Am J Roentgenol 165:125–133

CT and MR to Assess the Response of Liver Tumors to Hepatic Perfusion

M. Prokop

Medizinische Hochschule Hannover, Carl-Neuberg-Strasse 1, D-30625 Hannover, Germany

Abstract

Assessment of the response of liver tumors to hepatic perfusion is strongly based on cross-sectional imaging. CT and MRI have gained considerably in diagnostic accuracy with the introduction of new, fast acquisition techniques such as spiral CT or breath-hold techniques in MRI. In addition, the administration of contrast agents has improved and has led to new injection protocols in spiral CT and the development of liver-specific contrast agents in MRI. Imaging techniques, however, strongly rely on changes in morphology such as size, vascularization and signs of necrosis. Functional signs of tumor metabolism cannot be visualized directly. While most functional imaging techniques at present are based on nuclear medicine, MR spectroscopy (MRS) offers the potential to assess tumor metabolism. Its promise is a direct match between the morphologic information of MRI and the metabolic information provided by MRS. The application of MRS to the liver, however, is still in its infancy. This article will give an overview of the multitude of CT and MR techniques that can be used to monitor tumor response. It will discuss the various signs of tumor regression and some typical complications of hepatic perfusion therapy. In particular, the influence of tumor characteristics on the optimum choice of imaging technique will be demonstrated.

Introduction

For assessment of tumor response to hepatic perfusion, imaging techniques are considered the diagnostic standard since they are able to demonstrate direct signs of tumor regression (Table 1) as well as potential complications. However, they are strongly based on morphology. Since positive response to therapy does not necessarily lead to complete regression of macroscopic lesions, tumor metabolism should be considered as well. While serum tumor markers (if available) give an indication of overall tumor activity, it may be important to match serological markers with signs of local tumor activity in the liver. Most functional imaging techniques, such as single photon com-

Recent Results in Cancer Research, Vol. 147

Table 1. Main morphological signs of positive response to therapy

- Decrease of tumor size
- Direct signs of tumor necrosis
- Decrease of tumor vascularization as an indicator of decreased tumor vitality
- Formation of scar tissue

puted tomography (SPECT) and positron emission tomography (PET), are based on nuclear medicine. There are, however, MR-based techniques that use MR spectroscopy (MRS) to assess tumor metabolism. The main promise is a direct match between the morphological information of MRI and the metabolic information provided by MRS. While MRS is being introduced to in vivo assessment of tumor metabolism in the brain, its application to the liver is still in its infancy.

This article will give an overview of the multitude of CT and MR techniques that can be used to monitor tumor response. It will discuss the various signs of tumor regression and some typical complications of hepatic perfusion therapy. In particular, the influence of tumor characteristics on the optimum choice of imaging technique will be demonstrated.

MR Spectroscopy

Nuclear magnetic resonance spectroscopy was used to analyze biochemical substances in vitro long before MRI was introduced into clinical practice.

MRS offers an in vivo method to estimate the concentrations of various metabolic compounds within a three-dimensional tissue sample in the human body. There are a number of isotopes that lend themselves to MRS. The most abundant isotope, which also forms the basis for MRI, is the proton (^{1}H). In the liver, however, this isotope has not been used to analyze metabolic activity. Instead, ^{31}P spectroscopy and ^{19}F spectroscopy have been suggested (e.g., Henriksen 1994). ^{31}P spectroscopy allows for estimation of concentrations of ATP and other phosphorus metabolites originating from the energy metabolism of normal and tumor tissue. ^{19}F spectroscopy has been suggested to monitor the uptake of 5-fluorouracil (5-FU) into liver tumors (Murphy-Boesch et al. 1996).

Currently, simultaneous 3D acquisition of ^{31}P spectroscopy and ^{19}F spectroscopy is possible. The acquisition volume is subdivided into a $8 \times 8 \times 8$ matrix. The volume of each element ('voxel') is 64 ml. Acquisition time is 40 min, total examination time, 90 min (Gonen et al. 1996).

Typical findings for hepatic tumors include an increase in phosphomono- and phosphodiesters (PME and PDE) and an increase in the ratio between PME and β-ATP (Brinkmann and Melchert 1992; Cox et al. 1992; Schilling et al. 1992). After therapy, both an increase in PME and a decrease in PME and ATP have been reported (Cox et al. 1992; Saeki et al. 1992; Schilling et al. 1992). While some initial results are promising, the technique is only suited

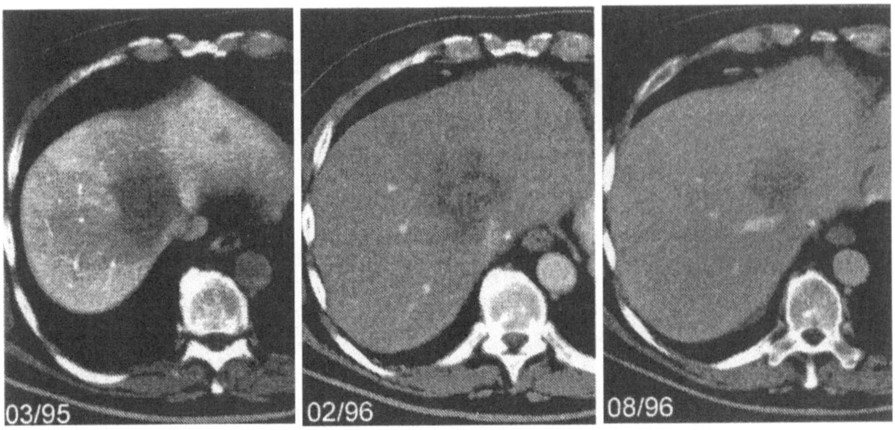

Fig. 1 a–c. Patient with metastasis from colorectal cancer. Compared to the CTAP study 1 month prior to hepatic perfusion therapy with mitomycin (**a**), the tumor size remained constant 10 months after treatment (**b**) but 6 months later decreased without further therapy (**c**)

for monitoring of relatively large tumors. It can be expected to be helpful in those cases in which there is initially neither regression nor progression in tumor size ('stable disease'; Fig. 1).

At present, however, the technique can be considered merely experimental, since technical requirements are high and acquisition time is too long to be practicable. Further drawbacks are the low spatial resolution and the shifting of the volume of interest during respiration. In addition, it is not proven whether vital tumor and the periphery of a lesion will be picked up in the presence of a necrotic center. As a result, a broader introduction of this technique into clinical routine cannot be expected in the near future.

Contrast Agents for CT and MRI

The detection rates for hepatic tumors in CT scans without administration of contrast medium are rather low (50-60%), depending on tumor histology and tumor size (Bernardino et al. 1986). In MRI, the detection rate is higher (60-80%; Wernecke et al. 1991; Hamm et al. 1997); however, the tumor size is often not displayed correctly.

With use of contrast agents (Helmberger et al. 1993; Liou et al. 1994; Yamamoto et al. 1995; Kuszyk et al. 1996; Urhahn et al. 1996), both detection rate and tumor depiction are significantly improved in CT and MRI (sensitivity up to 95%).

One can distinguish between interstitial contrast agents and liver-specific contrast agents. Interstitial contrast agents first pass the vascular system, then the liver parenchyma, and later diffuse into the liver interstitium. Liver-specific contrast agents are incorporated into normal hepatic cells (Kupffer cells or hepatocytes).

Interstitial Contrast Agents

Interstitial contrast agents are the basis of most standard techniques for CT and MR imaging of the liver. Interstitial contrast agents lead to a time-dependent liver-to-lesion contrast and allow for assessment of the tumor perfusion. In CT, all commercially available contrast agents are iodine-based interstitial agents. In MR, interstitial agents were the first compounds to be introduced into clinical practice. All interstitial MR agents are based on gadolinium (Gd) compounds.

With injection of interstitial contrast agents, three phases of contrast enhancement in the liver are distinguished: the arterial, the portal venous and the interstitial (or equilibrium) phase. Dependent on whether lesions are hypervascular or hypovascular (Table 2), the results of the techniques vary with respect to lesion detection, characterization and volumetrics (Baron 1994).

In the *arterial phase*, the contrast agent arrives in the liver via the hepatic artery only (approximately 10-20 s after intravenous injection of the contrast agent) and leads to increased contrast of all regions that are hyperperfused relative to the liver parenchyma (Murakami et al. 1995; Bonaldi et al. 1995a).

In the *portal venous phase*, the portal venous return of contrast material dominates. Since hepatic lesions (with the rare exception of some adenomas and well-differentiated hepatocellular carcinomas) are not perfused via the portal venous system, lesions appear hypointense relative to the surrounding parenchyma. Thus, this perfusion phase should be best suited for tumor detection and volumetrics. However, this holds true only for those techniques in which contrast material is entering the liver exclusively via the portal vein (arterioportal CT, or CTAP). With intravenous contrast application (standard techniques of contrast application in CT or MR), the effects of portal venous

Table 2. Summary of lesions according to perfusion

Hyperperfused lesions
HCC
Metastases of
• (Neuro-)endocrine tumors
• Renal cell carcinoma
• Malignant melanoma
• Sarcomas
Peripherally hyperperfused/hypoperfused lesions
CCC
Metastases of
• Colorectal cancer
• Other gastrointestinal tumors
• Breast cancer
• Bronchial carcinoma
• Sarcomas

enhancement of normal liver parenchyma and of arterial enhancement of tumors are superimposed: hypervascular lesions may be masked if the tumor hypervascularity matches the enhancement of liver parenchyma (Baron 1994). Due to the same effect, tumors with a hypervascular rim may appear smaller than they really are.

In the *interstitial phase*, the contrast material is diffused into the hepatic and tumor interstitium. Tumor necrosis is best detected in this phase, while the tumors themselves often can no longer be differentiated from normal liver parenchyma (Baron 1994).

Liver-specific Contrast Agents

While liver-specific contrast agents are still under development for CT, a number of compounds are already available for MR. One group (T2 agents) is based on superparamagnetic iron oxides (SPIO), which are taken up by the Kupffer cells and lead to a homogeneous decrease of signal intensity in T2-weighted images (Yamamoto et al. 1995; Vogl et al. 1994). The other group (T1 agents) are based on gadolinium or manganese compounds, which lead to a signal increase in the liver on T1-weighted images. Both types of contrast agents allow for improved liver-to-lesion contrast and markedly improve detection rates to between 80% and 95% (Vogl et al. 1994; Liou et al. 1994). Since there is high lesion contrast, volumetrics are improved after administration of contrast medium.

Computed Tomography

Computed tomography, still the most widely applied technique for liver imaging, has seen significant improvements in lesion detection and characterization with the advent of spiral CT. A multitude of scanning techniques are available (Table 3). The application of iodinated contrast agents is mandatory for most indications, including the monitoring of treatment response.

Table 3. Scanning techniques for liver CT

Technique	Remarks
• Pre-contrast scan	Useful adjunct for hypervascular lesions
Intravenous contrast administration	
• Contrast infusion	Obsolete
• Dynamic incremental CT	Inferior to spiral CT
• Spiral CT (portal venous phase)	Technique of choice for hypovascular lesions
• Biphasic spiral CT (arterial + portal phase)	Technique of choice for hypervascular lesions
Intraarterial contrast administration	
• CTAP, CTP	Highest sensitivity, artifact-prone
• Lipiodol CT	Only useful for hepatocellular carcinoma

Spiral CT Versus Standard CT

Data acquisition in standard CT is performed stepwise, section by section. Patients have to be able to constantly reproduce their inspirational depth for each of the 15-20 single scans necessary to acquire the whole liver. Breathing effects may lead loss of detection of smaller lesions or suboptimal display of larger lesions (Bonaldi et al. 1995b). Spiral CT allows for continuous volume acquisition within a relatively short time of 20-30 s. Examinations of the whole liver can be performed within one breath-hold phase. Thus, breathing effects are almost completely excluded. The detection rate is improved and volumetric measurements become more precise (Helmberger et al. 1995; Van Hoe et al. 1997).

Optimum display of lesions is strongly dependent on the technique of contrast application. Since 2-5 min are required to scan the whole liver with standard CT techniques, imaging in the arterial phase (which occurs 20-60 s after the beginning of intravenous contrast injection) is not possible. Only the portal venous phase can be used for interpretation. The scanning procedure has to be as fast as possible: small lesions may be masked due to diffusion of contrast into the periphery of lesions. If one waits too long, lesions may appear smaller than they really are. The detection rate is 60-70% with optimum technique (Wernecke et al. 1991). Hyperperfused lesions are often missed since they tend to take up contrast (due to arterial hyperperfusion) in a way similar to liver parenchyma (via portal venous perfusion).

In spiral CT, imaging is possible both in the arterial and the portal venous phase. Detection rates with i.v. contrast application rise to 80-90% (Murakami et al. 1995; Kuszyk et al. 1996).

Biphasic CT

Biphasic CT is a technique that scans the liver in both the arterial and the portal venous phase. Biphasic scans can only be performed with spiral technique since the arterial phase lasts only some 20–40 s. It is the arterial phase, however, in which most tumors show up that are missed on 'standard' portal venous images. Additionally, the arterial phase can be employed to estimate the amount of devascularization that occurs as a response to therapy. Since there is the potential to differentiate hemangiomas and focal nodular hyperplasia from malignant lesions, the technique can be used to increase the specificity of CT in determining response to therapy.

Biphasic CT is the recommended technique for liver imaging whenever optimum follow-up is required and it is not known whether a lesion is arterially hyper- or hypoperfused. While arterial phase imaging is helpful for hepatocellular carcinoma (Murakami et al. 1995) and hypervascular metastases (Table 2), portal venous imaging is sufficient for colorectal or breast cancer metastases (Kuszyk et al. 1996).

Arterioportal CT

Arterioportal CT (CTAP) has the highest sensitivity for lesion detection (>90%) when combined with spiral technique (Helmberger et al. 1993). Also, size measurements are most accurate with this technique independent of whether a lesion is hypo- or hyperperfused. There are two main drawbacks: The technique requires placement of an arterial catheter in the superior mesenteric or splenic artery (indirect portography), which is generally too great an effort for follow-up. In addition, compression or occlusion of portal venous branches will lead to wedge-shaped perfusion defects that make evaluation of these areas impossible. Thus, CTAP is not a suitable technique for monitoring therapy effects after liver perfusion.

Portal CT

Portal CT (CTP) is a variant of CTAP that requires placement of a portal venous port system: a port or pump system is implanted subcutaneously with a catheter that ends in the superior mesenteric vein or portal vein. Administration of diluted contrast material (< 150 mg/ml) will lead to an immediate contrast enhancement of the portal venous system (Fig. 2).

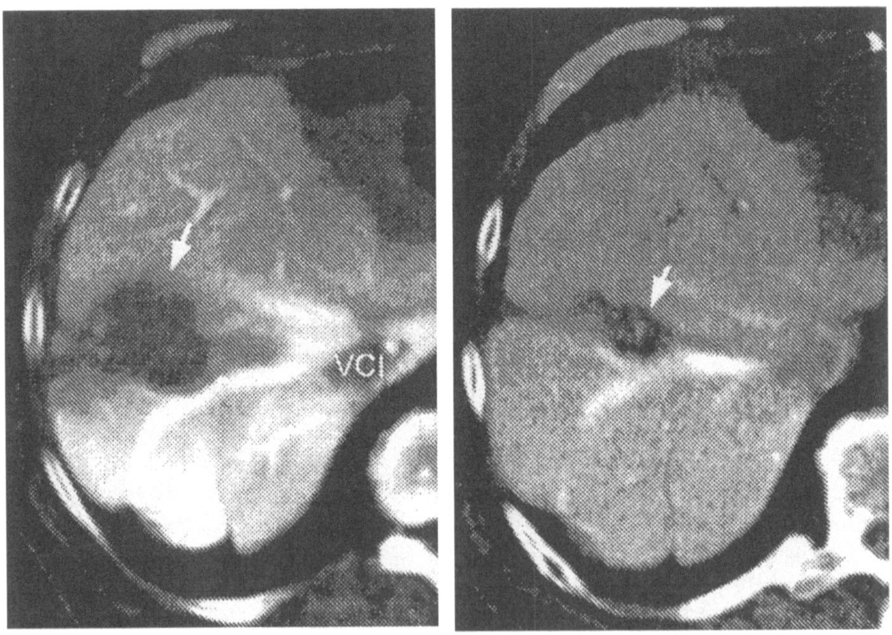

a b

Fig. 2 a, b. Patient with metastasis from colorectal cancer after regional tumor therapy. Comparison of CTP scans (obtained by injecting contrast agent via a portal venous port catheter) 3 months (**a**) and 9 months (**b**) after initiation of therapy. The large lesion in segment 8 was significantly reduced in size, and a narrow, hypodense scar formed that led to an indentation of the liver surface

This is a very suitable technique given that such a device is implanted during surgery. The main prerequisite, however, is that tumors do not compress portal venous branches. In practice this can be assumed if single tumor nodules are small. With small section thickness, tumor volumetrics can be performed very well. In larger tumors, however, the technique is artifact-prone.

Magnetic Resonance Imaging

MRI has suffered from marked variations in image quality between examinations even with identical scanning parameters. Some images are excellent, while others suffer from motion artifacts (breathing, pulsation) despite various measures for artifact suppression. Only with the advent of new breath-hold sequences have these artifacts been reduced sufficiently to make MRI a suitable technique for follow-up after therapy (Hamm et al. 1994, 1997; De Lange et al. 1994; Siewert et al. 1994).

There is no general rule as to which scan sequence yields the best results (Table 4). In scanners with medium to low field strength ($\leq$0.5 T), T1-weighted images tend to be best suited to display the lesions. In high-field magnets ($\geq$1 T), moderately T2-weighted sequences are to be preferred. Given optimized breath-hold sequences, the injection of interstitial Gd contrast agents does not improve lesion detection or characterization.

Table 4. Scanning techniques for liver MR

Technique	Remarks
• Pre-contrast MR	Best results with breath-hold techniques
Interstitial agents (Gd)	
• Post-Gd MR	No advantage as compared to breath-hold MR
• Dynamic MR	Improved results for hypervascular lesions
Liver-specific agents	
• SPIO (iron oxides)	Good technique for volumetrics (breath-hold MR)
• Gd-EOB	Good lesion contrast (volumetrics)
• Mn-DPDP	Good lesion contrast (volumetrics)

Spin-echo Sequences

Spin-echo (SE) techniques are characterized by large section thickness (7–8 mm), moderate to high lesion contrast, a moderate detection rate (60–70%) and strong vulnerability to breathing artifacts. However, if patient cooperation is good, a consistently high image quality can be obtained (Fig. 3). Recent technical improvements (e.g., fast SE) have considerably reduced acqui-

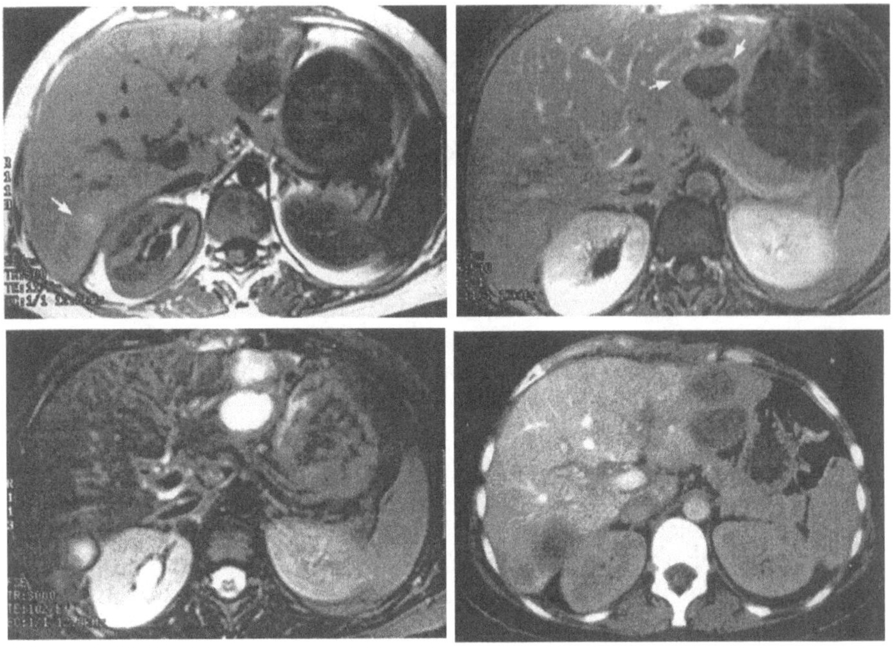

Fig. 3 a–d. Patient with metastasis from colorectal carcinoma after perfusion with mitomycin: comparison of various MR sequences and spiral CT. Tumor nodes appear hypointense on T1-weighted MR images; the central hemorrhage in a metastasis in segment 6 is typically hyperintense (arrow) (**a**). On a fat-suppressed image after intravenous application of Gd (as an interstitial contrast agent), there is minimum peripheral perfusion of the tumors in the left lateral segment (slight signal increase). The central hypodense region is typical for tumor necrosis (**b**). On a T2-weighted image, necrosis and hemorrhage appear hyperintense (**c**). A corresponding spiral CT image (portal venous phase) shows hypodense areas compatible with necrosis (**d**)

sition time, but breath-hold techniques are generally not yet possible. SE techniques will therefore mainly serve as an adjunct to other techniques.

Gradient-echo Sequences

Gradient-echo (GRE) techniques are characterized by large section thickness, moderate to high lesion contrast, breath-hold imaging, and a good detection rate that depends on contrast application and the (T1/T2) weighting of the sequence. Since it is fast and reliable, GRE is at present the MR technique of choice for follow-up.

Interstitial Contrast Agents

In contrast to CT, interstitial contrast agents (e.g., Gd-DTPH, Magnevist) do not improve lesion detection as compared to pre-contrast MR scans if modern scanners with breath-hold sequences are employed (Hamm et al. 1997).

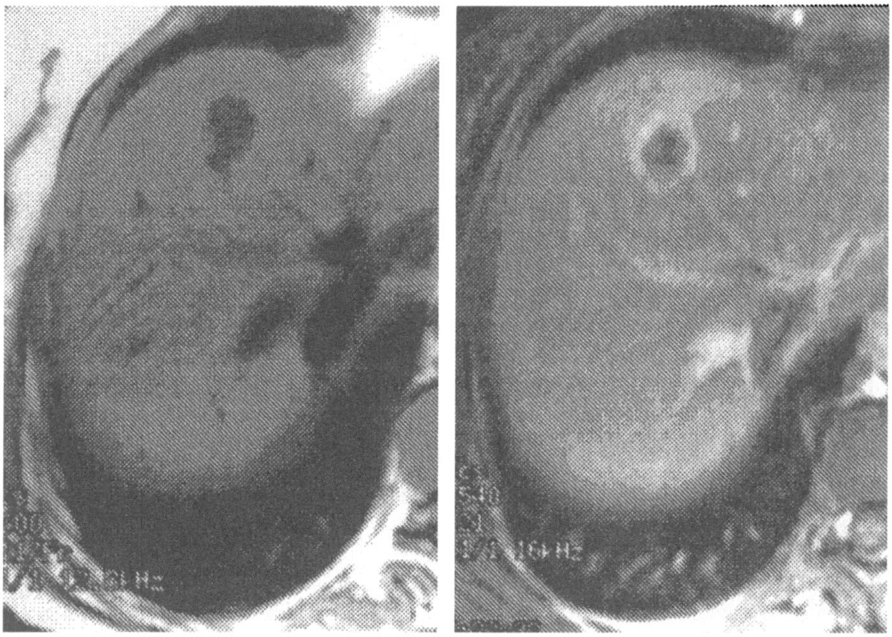

a b

Fig. 4a, b. Patient with metastasis from a colorectal carcinoma after perfusion with mitomycin. While the standard T1-weighted MR image only showed a hypodense lesions consistent with necrosis (**a**), the fat-suppressed image after intravenous application of Gd demonstrated residual tumor perfusion in the lesion periphery (**b**)

In hypervascular tumors, however, dynamic sequences that acquire images in the arterial as well as the portal venous phase may further improve lesion detection and characterization similar to biphasic spiral CT (Murakami et al. 1995). MR sequences that use additional fat suppression eliminate the high signal from subcutaneous and intraabdominal fat. Thus, high signal only is due to regions of increased contrast uptake after Gd administration. Dynamic sequences with fat suppression are therefore particularly helpful for assessment of tumor vascularization as a measure of response to therapy (Fig. 4).

Liver-specific Contrast Agents

Liver-specific contrast agents further improve lesion detection with MRI. Since tumor-to-liver contrast is particularly high, these agents are well suited for volumetric measurements. However, there is a substantial cost increase when such agents are used.

Monitoring of Treatment Response

Choice of Lesions for Monitoring Therapy Response

Since a multitude of artifacts can interfere with adequate visualization of lesions, one should try to choose lesions that are both representative for the disease and visualized well enough to be suitable for follow-up. Usually, lesions smaller than 2 cm cannot be considered appropriate for follow-up of therapy response since their detection is excessively subject to breathing artifacts and partial volume effects.

Partial volume effects are the more apparent the smaller the lesions are relative to the chosen section thickness. If a single volume element (voxel) within the data set does not correspond to only one type of tissue, CT numbers or MR signal intensities will be influenced by all tissues within the voxel. Thus, lesion contrast will be diminished and lesions may appear smaller than they are.

Respiratory movements during a scan (non-breath-hold MRI scans) will lead to artifacts; variations in inspiratory depth (standard CT) will lead to inconstant depiction or even loss of lesions. MR is especially dependent on patient cooperation, since breathing artifacts may completely ruin the image.

Tumor Size

Tumor size is the most useful criterion for follow-up. For the determination of tumor response (according to WHO criteria), the two largest diameters that are perpendicular to each other have to be determined from axial images. This, however, is a rather crude parameter for follow-up. The determination of tumor volumes is much more accurate (see below).

Tumor size may fail as an indicator of positive response to therapy if central necrosis develops without apparent decrease in tumor size. In most cases, however, central tumor necrosis will eventually be followed by size reduction (Fig. 5). Reduction in tumor size is thus not an early indicator of therapy success, and in some cases with slow tumor regression, only the criteria for 'stable disease' will be met between consecutive follow-up examinations (Fig. 1).

Tumor Volumetrics

Prerequisites for tumor volumetrics are sufficient tumor-to-liver contrast, a sufficiently large tumor relative to the section thickness, and the absence of movement artifacts (Helmberger et al. 1995). Appropriate software can be used to digitally measure tumor volume.

In simple cases, tumor volume can be estimated by an ellipsoid. For this purpose, the largest lesion diameter a has to be determined. Then, the larg-

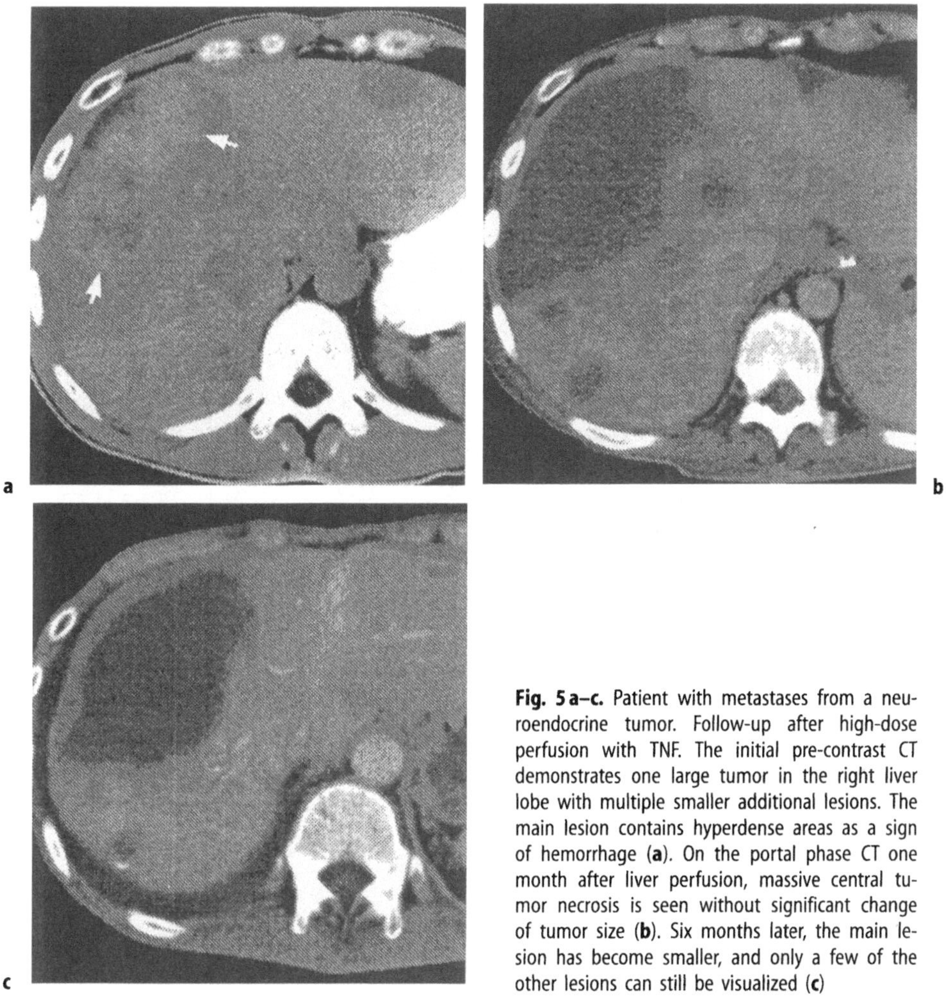

Fig. 5 a–c. Patient with metastases from a neuroendocrine tumor. Follow-up after high-dose perfusion with TNF. The initial pre-contrast CT demonstrates one large tumor in the right liver lobe with multiple smaller additional lesions. The main lesion contains hyperdense areas as a sign of hemorrhage (**a**). On the portal phase CT one month after liver perfusion, massive central tumor necrosis is seen without significant change of tumor size (**b**). Six months later, the main lesion has become smaller, and only a few of the other lesions can still be visualized (**c**)

est diameter *b* that is perpendicular to *a* has to be found. Finally, the largest remaining diameter *c* that is both perpendicular to *a* and *b* has to be measured. Tumor volume *V* can then be estimated by the simple formula: $V=(a+b+c)/2$.

In more complex lesions that do not have a convex contour, slice by slice measurements of tumor area *A* have to be performed using software that is available on most scanners or workstations. The resulting volume *V* can determined by adding up all measured areas on the cross-sectional images and multiplying it by the distance between adjacent sections. Since this task may be cumbersome, newer volumetric software is available that simplifies this approach by providing automatic detection of boundaries (Fig. 6) and automatic calculation of the resulting tumor volume (Helmberger et al. 1995; van

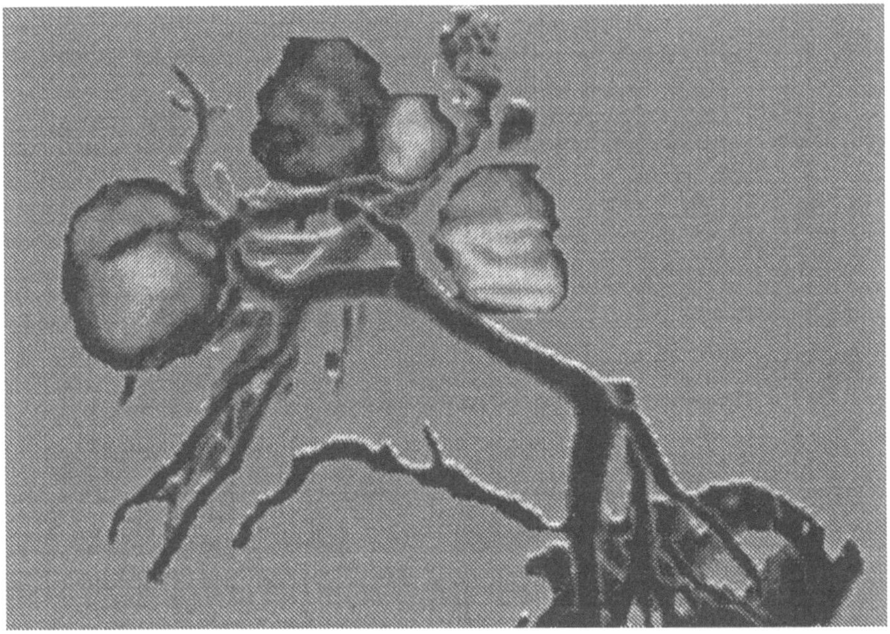

Fig. 6. Volumetric display of multiple liver metastases obtained from a spiral CTAP data set by using computer-aided visualization techniques (shaded surface display after data editing using region growing algorithms)

Hoe et al. 1997). A fully automated approach, however, is limited if tumor-to-liver contrast is low.

Tumor Perfusion

In the arterial perfusion phase, tumors display various perfusion patterns depending on their histology and treatment response (Table 2). Most hyperperfused lesions are hepatocellular carcinomas or metastases of endocrine tumors or of renal cell carcinoma. Cholangiocellular carcinomas and metastases of many tumors, including colorectal and breast cancer, present as peripherally hyperperfused lesions that are characterized by a typical rim enhancement in the arterial phase. The same tumors may also be hypoperfused, and then cannot be detected on arterial phase images. Even these tumors, however, will eventually take up some contrast in the portal venous phase, but much less so than the surrounding liver parenchyma. Thus they will appear hypointense relative to the normal liver.

Positive response to treatment generally leads to a reduction in tumor perfusion. This is most easily observed in hyperperfused lesions. These lesions may be transformed into peripherally hyperperfused or hypoperfused lesions (Fig. 4). Both biphasic CT or dynamic MRI after injection of Gd contrast

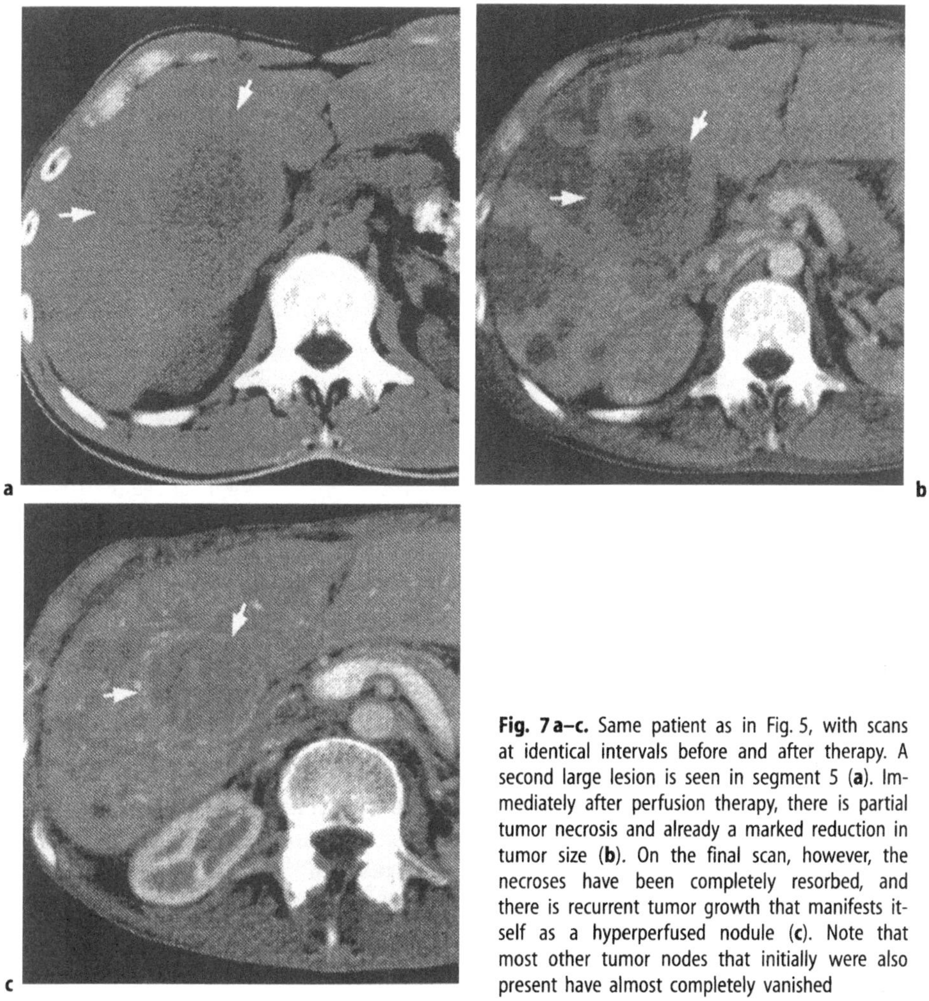

Fig. 7 a–c. Same patient as in Fig. 5, with scans at identical intervals before and after therapy. A second large lesion is seen in segment 5 (**a**). Immediately after perfusion therapy, there is partial tumor necrosis and already a marked reduction in tumor size (**b**). On the final scan, however, the necroses have been completely resorbed, and there is recurrent tumor growth that manifests itself as a hyperperfused nodule (**c**). Note that most other tumor nodes that initially were also present have almost completely vanished

agents can be used to observe these effects. Tumor necrosis results in areas that no longer take up contrast, either in the arterial or in the portal perfusion phase (Figs. 4, 5, 7).

Tumor Necrosis

In CT, tumor necrosis is characterized by a hypodense lesion (near-water density: 0–30 HU) that does not take up contrast (Figs. 3 5, 7). The difference in CT numbers between the pre- and post-contrast scans should be less than 10 HU.

In MR, tumor necrosis exhibits the typical signs of protein-rich fluids: it has a high signal on T2-weighted images (similar to spinal fluid) but may have low to high signal intensities on T1-weighted images (depending on whether there is hemorrhage or not; cf. Fig. 3). Again, there is no contrast uptake on the post-contrast scans (Fig. 4).

Residual Tumor

Residual tumor is seen most often in the periphery of a treated lesion. In hepatic perfusion therapy, it may be more frequent with aberrant arterial supply. In contrast to tumor recurrence, residual tumor is present on the first control examination after perfusion therapy.

Recurrent Tumor

Recurrent tumor is characterized by new tumor nodules or recurrent growth of a seemingly inactive lesion. After hepatic perfusion therapy it is most often seen in the periphery of a treated lesion. There may be initial shrinking of the lesion (e.g., resorption of central necrosis) despite recurrent tumor growth (Fig. 6).

Scarring

Scarring, cysts or restitution represent the final results of successful therapy. In CT, hepatic scars appear as hypodense, bandlike structures in areas of former tumor activity (Fig. 2). On MR, older scars are hypointense on T2-weighted images. With either technique, scars tend to take up contrast slowly. Contrast enhancement is often most pronounced in the interstitial phase.

Imaging of Complications

There is a multitude of potential complications (Table 5) that may be picked up either by CT or MRI. The most comprehensive imaging technique for this purpose is biphasic spiral CT, since it allows for imaging both of soft tissues and of the relevant vascular structures.

Choice of Examination Technique for Follow-up

Since tumor size is the most important indicator of therapy success, the examination technique for follow-up has to be chosen accordingly. The conspicuity of various tumor entities often cannot be accurately predicted for the various scanning techniques. If more than one technique was available preoperatively, the one with the best lesion contrast and the least artifacts

Table 5. Complications after hepatic perfusion therapy

Complications secondary to chemotherapy
• Liver necrosis
• Arterial occlusion
• Portal venous occlusion
• Budd Chiari
• Infection/abscess formation
Complications secondary to operative approach
• Hematoma
• Bleeding
• Vessel damage (e.g., dissection, thrombosis)
• Direct organ injury
• Infection

Table 6. Choice of imaging technique for follow-up after hepatic perfusion therapy

Technique	Hypovascular lesions	Hypervascular lesions	Volumetrics	Artifacts/ reproducibility	Invasiveness	Cost
CT	+	–	+/–	(+)	++	+
Spiral CT (portal)	+	++	+/–	++	++	+
Biphasic CT	++	++	++	++	++	++
CTAP	++	++	++	–	–	–
CTP	++	++	++	–	+	+
MRI	+	+/–	+/–	+/–	++	+/–
MRI (breath-hold)	+	++	+	++	++	+/–
MRI (+Gd)	++	++	+	+	++	–
MRI (liver-specific)	++	++	++	++	++	–

++= Very good; + = good; +/– = mixed; – = problematic

should be selected for follow-up. If one is free to chose the examination technique, Table 6 gives an overview of which one is best suited in a particular setting.

In general, portal phase spiral CT will be the best choice for follow-up of hypovascular lesions such as colorectal metastases (in terms of tumor contrast, reproducibility, lack of artifacts, and costs), while either biphasic spiral CT or breath-hold MRI should be chosen for hypervascular lesions such as metastases from renal carcinoma. If cost is no issue, current data suggest that breath-hold MRI with liver-specific contrast agents will yield the best results. CTAP, although highly accurate in smaller lesions, is too invasive (angiography required) and is artifact-prone in larger lesions.

Discussion

MRS for monitoring of therapy response after perfusion of liver tumors is far from entering clinical practice. There is, however, growing evidence that MRS may be feasible for monitoring therapy response in larger lesions even if the lesion does not completely occupy the volume of interest used to determine ^{31}P spectra (Saeki et al. 1992). MRS of ^{19}F spectra may be helpful to directly monitor the metabolism of 5-FU during or after chemotherapy.

Since only lesions larger than 2 cm are reproducible enough to be relevant for follow-up, choice of imaging technique is not as critical as in presurgical work-up. Whatever technique (scan protocol and method of contrast administration) has been chosen, however, should be continued throughout the evaluation period in the same patient.

If CT is chosen, the spiral technique should be obligatory, since even larger lesions may be underestimated on standard CT if inspiratory depth varies between sections. Biphasic CT in the arterial and portal venous phase is the technique of choice for hypervascular lesions and for imaging of complications. A single spiral scan in the portal venous phase is simpler but should be employed only in hypovascular tumors (as determined from the pre-treatment scans); in the case of hypervascular or peripherally hypervascular lesions, tumor size may be underestimated. CTP can be a suitable and highly accurate alternative in patients in whom a port catheter has been implanted into the portal or superior mesenteric vein. This, however, requires intraoperative placement of such a device and may be complicated by venous thrombosis or dislocation of the port catheter.

MRI is even more dependent upon optimum technology than CT. Breath-hold (GRE) sequences should always be included in the MR study. Gadolinium as an interstitial contrast agent may only be helpful in selected cases if dynamic MR studies are performed during various perfusion phases. Liver-specific contrast agents appear to be well suited for follow-up and tumor volumetrics; however, they are still rather expensive.

With respect to follow-up, tumor size is the most useful morphologic criterion but may fail if there is marked central necrosis or slow tumor regression (Fig. 1). Tumor vascularization is mostly helpful in hypervascular lesions. Here, reduction of hyperperfused areas may be the first sign of tumor response to treatment. Tumor necrosis is a relatively rare finding that is mostly seen in the acute phase after liver perfusion. Residual tumor or tumor recurrence are seen most often in the periphery of lesions. Complications from liver perfusion are readily apparent on both CT and MRI, with biphasic CT superior for the demonstration of arterial complications.

In general, spiral CT and (non-contrast-enhanced) MRI (breath-hold GRE sequences) appear to be similarly suitable imaging techniques in following up liver lesions after hepatic perfusion therapy.

References

Baron RL (1994) Understanding and optimizing use of contrast material for CT of the liver. AJR 163:323-331

Bernardino ME, Erwin BC, Steinberg HV, et al (1986) Delayed hepatic CT scanning: increased confidence and improved detection of hepatic metastases. Radiology 159:71-74

Bonaldi VM, Bret PM, Reinhold C, Atri M (1995a) Comparison of helical and conventional computed tomography of the liver. Can Assoc Radiol J, 46:443-448

Bonaldi VM, Bret PM, Reinhold C, Atri M (1995b) Helical CT of the liver: value of an early hepatic arterial phase. Radiology 197:357-363

Brinkmann G, Melchert UH (1992) A study of T1-weighted 31phosphorus MR-spectroscopy from patients with focal and diffuse liver disease. Magn Reson Imaging 10:949-956

Cox IJ, Menon DK, Sargentoni J, et al (1992) Phosphorus-31 magnetic resonance spectroscopy of the human liver using chemical shift imaging techniques. J Hepatol 14:265-275

De Lange EE, Mugler JP, Bosworth JE, et al (1994) Imaging of the liver: breath hold T1 weighted MP-GRE compared with conventional T2 weighted SE MR imaging - lesion detection, localization and characterization. Radiology 190:727-736

Gonen O, Li C, Murphy-Boesch J, et al (1996) Simultaneous 3D chemical imaging of H-1 decoupled F-19 and P-31 in human liver during chemotherapy. Radiology 192(P):428

Hamm B, Thoeni RF, Gould RG, et al (1994) Focal liver lesions: characterization with nonenhanced and dynamic contrast material-enhanced MR imaging. Radiology 190:417-424

Hamm B, Mahfouz AE, Taupitz M, et al (1997) Liver metastases: improved detection with dynamic Gd-enhanced MR imaging. Radiology 202:677-682

Helmberger H, Bautz W, Vogel U, Lenz M (1993) CT-Arterioportographie in Spiraltechnik zum Nachweis von Lebermetastasen. Rofo 158:410-415

Helmberger H, Bautz W, Sendler A, Fink U, Gerhardt P (1995) Volumetrie abdomineller Tumoren. Problemstellung - Lösungsansätze. Radiologe 35:587-591

Henriksen O (1994) MR spectroscopy in clinical research. Acta Radiol 35:96-116

Kuszyk BS, Bluemke DA, Urban BA, et al (1996) Portal-phase contrast-enhanced helical CT for the detection of malignant hepatic tumors: sensitivity based on comparison with intraoperative and pathologic findings. AJR 166:91-95

Liou J, Lee JK, Borrello JA, Brown JJ (1994) Differentiation of hepatomas from nonhepatomatous masses: use of MnDPDP-enhanced MR images. Magn Reson Imaging 12:71-79

Murakami T, Kim T, Oi H, et al (1995) Detectability of hypervascular hepatocellular carcinoma by arterial phase images of MR and spiral CT. Acta Radiol 36:372-376

Murphy-Boesch J, Li C, He L, et al (1996) Proton-decoupled F-19 spectroscopy of 5-FU catabolites in human liver. Radiology 192(P):427

Saeki M, Ashida H, Imamura K, et al (1992) Clinical application of 31P MRS to malignant liver tumors-with an emphasis on evaluation of response to therapy. Nippon Igaku Hoshasen Gakkai Zasshi 52:744-754

Schilling A, Gewiese B, Berger G, et al (1992) Liver tumors: follow-up with P-31 MR spectroscopy after local chemotherapy and chemoembolization. Radiology 182:887-890

Siewert B, Müller MF, Foley M, Wielopolski PA, Finn JP (1994) Fast MR imaging of the liver: quantitative comparison of techniques. Radiology 193:37-42

Urhahn R, Adam G, Keulers P, Kilbinger M, Günther RW (1996) Erkennbarkeit fokaler Leberläsionen: Vergleich von MRT bei 1,5 T und dynamischer Spiral-CT. Rofo 164:301-307

Van Hoe L, Van Cutsem E, Vergote I, et al (1997) Size Quantification of liver metastases of patients undergoing cancer treatment: reproducibility of one, two and three-dimensional measurements determined with spiral CT. Radiology 202:671-676

Vogl TJ, Hammerstingl R, Pegios W, et al (1994) Wertigkeit des leberspezifischen superparamagnetischen Kontrastmittels AMI-25 für die Detektion und Differentialdiagnose lebereigener Tumoren versus Metastasen. Rofo 160:319-328

Wernecke K, Rummeny E, Bongartz G, et al (1991) Detection of hepatic masses in patients with carcinoma: comparative sensitivities of sonography, CT and MR imaging. AJR 157:731–739

Yamamoto K, Shimizu T, Hiraishi K, et al (1995) Evaluation of AMI-25 enhanced MR imaging and enhanced helical CT for liver tumors. Nippon Igaku Hoshasen Gakkai Zasshi 55(1):1–6

VI. Future Aspects

Implications of Heat Shock Proteins During Liver Surgery and Liver Perfusion

Y. Yamamoto, M. Kume, and Y. Yamaoka

Department of Gastroenterological Surgery, Kyoto University, Graduate School of Medicine, 54 Kawahara-cho, Shogoin, Sakyo-ku, Kyoto 606-8397, Japan

Abstract

Cells primed by sublethal stress transiently overproduce heat shock proteins (HSPs) and thereby develop tolerance to the next lethal stress. This response in organisms is called the stress response and involves the induction of HSPs. To assist the liver in developing tolerance for warm ischemia-reperfusion injury, which sometimes jeopardizes the patients after extended surgery for malignancies with vascular invasion in the liver, basic experiments to activate the stress response using stress preconditioning were performed. Heat shock preconditioning in rat livers has been shown to induce tolerance against warm ischemia–reperfusion injury in normal, fibrotic, and steatotic livers. Ischemic preconditioning using short-term Pringle's maneuver and pharmacological preconditioning using doxorubicin were also effective. In rats, heat shock preconditioning protected livers from free radical injury induced by the oral administration of carbon tetrachloride. The above data were supported by animal survival, suppression of serum transaminase levels, and improved energy status of the liver after intervention. Increased production of HSP72 was observed after preconditioning. In addition, the significance of HSP production as a stress parameter was demonstrated during the reperfusion of congested portal blood to the ischemic liver. The ill effect of congested portal blood could not be detected by conventional parameters but was detected by observing the increase in HSP72 production. Stress preconditioning seems to be a promising strategy to counter the damaging effect of hepatic warm ischemia during liver surgery and liver perfusion.

Introduction

Liver resection techniques are well established and standardized for surgical treatment of liver cancer. The development of these surgical procedures has enabled us to perform liver resection safely in many cases. However, when liver cancer extends to the main branches of the portal or hepatic vein, the prognosis is still poor even after surgical intervention (Fig. 1). Manipulation

Recent Results in Cancer Research, Vol. 147

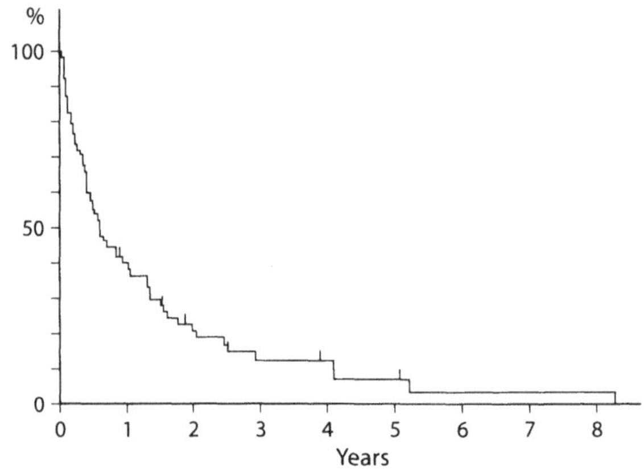

Fig. 1. Survival curve of 71 patients with hepatocellular carcinoma with tumor thrombi in the main branches of the portal vein, hepatic veins or both after hepatic resection between 1985 and 1995 in our department. Main branches of the portal vein include the first branch of the portal vein and the portal trunk and the main branches of the hepatic vein include the first branch of the hepatic vein and inferior vena cava. Complete tumor resection was performed in 72% of the patients and vascular reconstruction in 44%. The 3- and 5-year survivals were only 12.8% and 7.7%, respectively

of thrombi in the portal or hepatic vein easily results in multiple recurrence of the tumor in the remaining liver or lung. To prevent tumor dissemination downstream during manipulation, resection of the vessels with tumor thrombi intact and vascular reconstruction are necessary. When tumor invasion extends to the portal trunk or inferior vena cava, stopping blood inflow to the liver is necessary. The consequent hepatic ischemia-reperfusion injury is a matter of great importance because it essentially affects the patients' prognoses. *Ex situ* liver resection or *ex situ* storage of the remaining liver during complete resection of the tumor may help prevent intraoperative tumor dissemination. These techniques, however, also require the liver to tolerate a longer ischemic period.

The liver is reported to be more tolerant to portal triad clamping than has been previously considered (Huguet et al. 1992), and therefore the usefulness of Pringle's maneuver in liver surgery has been supported in Europe (Belghiti et al. 1996). The influence of ischemia-reperfusion injury is greater in patients with liver cirrhosis than in those with normal livers. In addition, unlike standard liver resection, the ischemic period is usually longer during operations that include vascular reconstruction, and the degree of transient reperfusion during vascular surgery cannot be predicted. The risk of postoperative liver failure therefore is regrettably high (Table 1).

To prevent cancer recurrence due to intraoperative dissemination during extended surgery in liver cancer patients with vascular invasion, the development of a strategy to assist the liver to tolerate ischemia-reperfusion injury is of great interest. Investigations to induce tolerance in cells or organs during unfavorable stress have been performed for the last decade (Lindquist 1986). In this field the acquisition of thermotolerance after heat shock stress

Table 1. Postoperative complications in HCC patients with tumor thrombi in the main branches of the portal or hepatic veins: 1985–1995

Complication	No. of patients (n=71)	No. of deaths
Liver failure	9	4
Intraabdominal bleeding	6	4
Intraabdominal infection	8	
Pleural effusion	8	
Massive ascites	5	
Sepsis	2	
Gastrointestinal bleeding	3	
Heart failure	1	1
Bile leakage	1	
Others	3	
Morbidity	49.2%	
Mortality	12.7%	

Some patients had multiple complications.
Main portal branches include the first branch of the portal vein and the portal trunk. The main branches of the hepatic vein include the first branch of the hepatic vein and the inferior vena cava.

is the most well-known (Hahn et al. 1982; Yamamori and Yura 1982; Li 1983; Li et al. 1983). The thermotolerance phenomenon has been observed in a broad range of organisms at various stages of development and on cultured cells grown under many conditions. Evidence suggests that the synthesis of heat shock proteins (HSPs) is the crucial element in the stress response (McAlister and Finkelstein 1980; Landry et al. 1982; Li et al. 1983; Velazquez and Lindquist 1984). Later studies using mostly cultured cells revealed that the protective effect of HSPs is not only beneficial toward thermal stress but for the most part, leads to improved resistance of the organism to enviromental stress (Polla 1988; Welch 1992). This phenomenon is known as cross-tolerance (Finnell et al. 1993). Hence it seems likely that by activating the stress response (preconditioning), tolerance against ischemia–reperfusion injury will result.

Results of the induction of tolerance to ischemia–reperfusion injury in rat livers by preconditioning and the possible participation of HSP72 in the development of this tolerance are discussed herein. HSPs are stress-activated proteins, and their significance as stress parameters after liver perfusion is discussed to illustrate the influence of congested portal blood to the ischemic liver. In addition, the preliminary results of HSP72 in human livers and liver cancer are introduced, and our perspective on the study of HSPs during liver perfusion therapy for liver cancer is discussed.

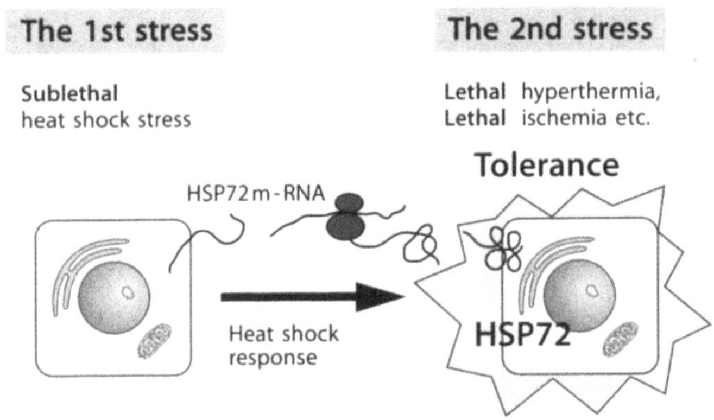

Fig. 2. Stress response and heat shock protein (HSP). Cells primed by sublethal stress transiently overproduced HSPs and developed tolerance to the next lethal stress

Stress Response

Living organisms respond to a variety of stressful situations by rapidly and transiently accelerating the production of specific proteins. A great deal of circumstantial evidence supports the belief that the function of these proteins is to protect cells from the ill effects of stress so the cells can recover and survive. The discovery of this phenomenon dates back to the discovery of "puff" formation in the chromosome of the salivary gland of *Drosophila* after heat shock exposure (Ritossa 1962). The significance of puff formation had been unclear until 1974 when Tissieres et al. discovered a small number of specific proteins produced upon puff formation, advancing the study of this phenomen. Since 1978 many investigations have revealed that a wide variety of organisms produce similar kinds of proteins after heat shock, and the term "heat shock protein" resulted (Lindquist 1986). Since 1977 many reports have described stressors other than heat shock that induce a similar response to the organism, including ischemia (Thaddeus and Nowak 1985), oxidative stress (Ohtsuki et al. 1992), and exposure to heavy metals (Heikkila et al. 1986), denatured proteins (Hightower 1980; Ananthan et al. 1986), amino acid analogues (Kelly and Schlesinger 1978), arsenite (Levinson et al. 1980), and bacterial toxins (Hensler et al. 1991). The response was thus not specific to heat shock stress, and so the new term "stress protein" was initiated. The terms HSP and stress protein are used interchangeably. At any rate, cells transiently overproduce HSPs in response to sublethal stress, thereby increasing their tolerance to the next potentially lethal stress (Fig. 2). The role of HSPs in the development of stress tolerance is therefore of great interest.

Heat Shock Proteins

Characterization of HSPs is not the focus of this article, and discussion of this subject may be found in the literature. In brief, these proteins have survived evolution and are found ubiquitously in a wide variety of organisms from bacteria to mammals (Bardwell and Craig 1984; Hunt and Morimoto 1985). The major HSPs have been classified into four families according to their molecular mass. The largest molecular mass group is called the HSP90 family; others are the HSP70 family, HSP60 family, and small HSPs. Some larger HSPs (about 100–110 kDa) with properties that differ from those of the other families have been identified in mammalian cells.

Proteins of the HSP70 family exist even within nonstress environments. These proteins are considered to have a pivotal role in the formation of tertiary structures by the folding of synthesized proteins, penetration of proteins through organelle membranes, assembly and disassembly of proteins, and decomposition of proteins. Based on the functions of HSP70, the term "molecular chaperone" (Ellis 1990) is used. HSP70 in eukaryocytes constitutes a multigene family consisting of several isotypes. HSP70, which is transiently produced depending on the stress attack, is called inducible-type HSP70, or HSP72. HSP72 has been proved to be this type of protein in the HSP70 family. Another HSP70, constitutively expressed in the cytosol and nucleus, is called heat shock cognate protein, or HSC70. Investigation has revealed that this protein is identical to HSP73 in the HSP70 family. Some other proteins of this family include GRP78, prp73, mtHSP70, and so on. Proteins of the HSP90 family always exist in the cytosol in relatively large amounts, and their relation with steroid hormones is well established. HSP90 exists in the cytosol as a dimer form and binds to steroid receptors. It is believed that this protein regulates the process by which steroid receptors bind to DNA. The HSP60 family is also called chaperonin 60. Proteins of this family function as molecular chaperones and exist mainly in mitochondria and chloroplasts in the eukaryocyte. HSP60 contributes to the maturity and complex formation of the mitochondrial proteins. Small-molecular-mass HSPs are HSP28, ubiquitin, and HSP47 among others.

Regulation of Heat Shock Genes

Although details of the regulatory mechanisms of HSPs have not yet been determined, a gene arrangement of heat shock element (HSE) has been discovered in the upper stream of the exon coding heat shock genes (Xiao and Lis 1988). Transcription of the heat shock gene begins when the heat shock factor (HSF) binds to HSE (Parker and Topol 1984). HSF is a protein consisting of 300–800 amino acids. The molecular weight of this factor differs among species, but HSPs are well conserved within the species. According to the theory of Morimoto et al. (1992), HSF usually exists assembled with HSP70. HSF in this form is considered to be inactive. When denatured proteins increase within the cytosol HSP70 mobilizes to react with the denatured proteins. On this occasion, HSF is disassembled from HSP70 and is activated to bind with HSE. When the amount of HSP including HSP70 increases, HSF reassembles with HSP70, and the facilitated transcription level returns to a regular level.

Stress Preconditioning of the Liver for Ischemia-Reperfusion Injury

Heat Shock Preconditioning

Many studies of HSPs have been done using cultured cells, particularly those of *Drosophila*. There are fewer trials, however, that investigate heat shock preconditioning *in vivo*, and only studies on isolated organs such as heart and kidneys exist (Currie 1987; Currie et al. 1988; Yellon et al. 1992).

In 1995 we studied the effects of whole-body heat shock preconditioning on the subsequent warm ischemia-reperfusion injury of the liver (Saad et al. 1995). Using the rats of the Wistar strain, body temperature was elevated to 42 °C for 15 min. Overexpression of messenger RNA coding HSP72 was de-

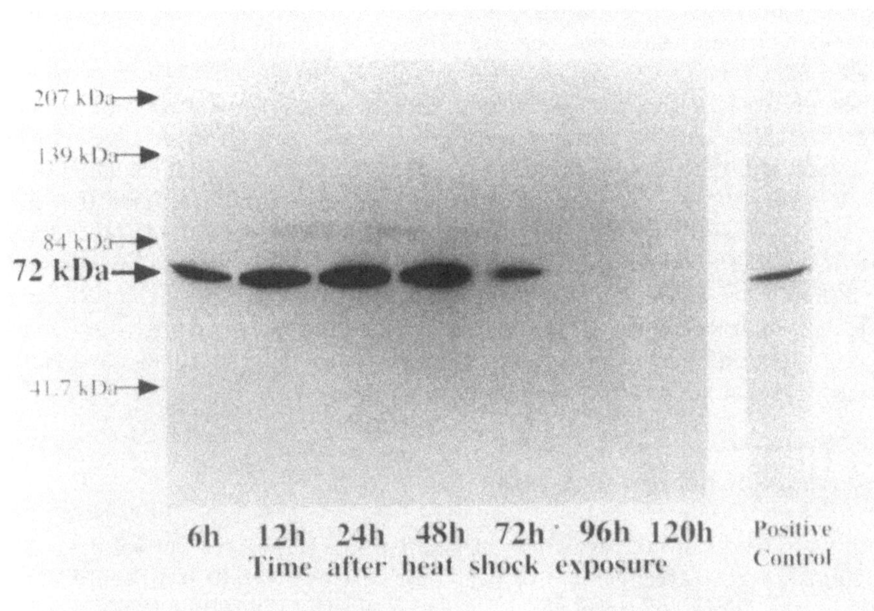

Fig. 3. Body temperatures were elevated to 42 °C for 15 min in Wistar rats. Rats were killed at specific times after heat shock preconditioning, and the production of HSP72 was analyzed by Western blot analysis using mouse antibody to HeLa cell HSP72. HSP72 accumulation increased from 6 h to 48 h after heat shock preconditioning and disappeared by 96 h. The protein concentrations were 3 μg/lane. The positive control is 0.2 μg/lane

tected in the liver immediately after heat shock preconditioning. The overexpression of messenger RNA had almost stopped 48 h after heat shock preconditioning. The production of HSP72 following this event is shown in Fig. 3. A Western blot test revealed that protein synthesis had started as early as 6 h after heat shock preconditioning, with peak production at 24–48 h after the initial event (Kume et al. 1996). The excess production of HSP72 protein had stopped within 96 h after preconditioning. Thus the effect of preconditioning to 30-min warm ischemia and reperfusion by portal triad clamping was tested. The survival rate on postoperative day 7 was better proportionally according to the amount of induced HSP72. The HSP72 production was at its maximal level 48 h after preconditioning. The 7-day survival of the animals after 30-min warm ischemic intervention at this point was 15 of 16 (93.8%) in the preconditioned group; in the control group only 8 of 16 (50%) had survived (Table 2). Differences in survival were supported by the early recovery of energy status and suppression of serum transaminase levels (Table 3).

Table 2. Survival of rats on postoperative day 7 after 30-min warm ischemia according to the intervals between heat shock preconditioning and ischemic load

Condition	Survival	
	No. of patients	%
Controls[a]	8/16	50
After ischemia		
24 h	15/16	94*
48 h	15/16	94*
72 h	14/16	88**
120 h	10/16	63

[a] Rats without heat shock preconditioning
* $P<0.01$ and ** $P<0.05$ compared with control by Kruskal-Wallis test ($n=16$)

Table 3. Biochemical parameters after 40 min of reperfusion following exposure to 30 min of warm ischemia

Parameter	Control	24 h	48 h	72 h	120 h
ALT	1229±450	695±141*	348±218*	429±146*	1284±369
LDH	14187±5547	6060±1838*	3534±1998*	5246±2095*	11673±2241
ATP	1.77±0.52	3.38±0.20*	3.08±0.26*	3.15±0.38*	2.27±0.55
EC	0.63±0.10	0.80±0.03*	0.78±0.03*	0.78±0.04*	0.69±0.10

Values are expressed as the mean ± SD
There were six subjects in each group
The intervals indicate how long after heat shock preconditioning the ischemic load was administered
Controls: those without heat shock preconditioning
ALT, serum alanine aminotransferase (IU/L); *LDH*, serum lactic dehydrogenase (IU/L); *ATP*, adenosine triphosphate level in tissue (µmol/g wet tissue weight); *EC*, energy charge potential of the liver
* $P<0.01$ compared with control by one-factor ANOVA

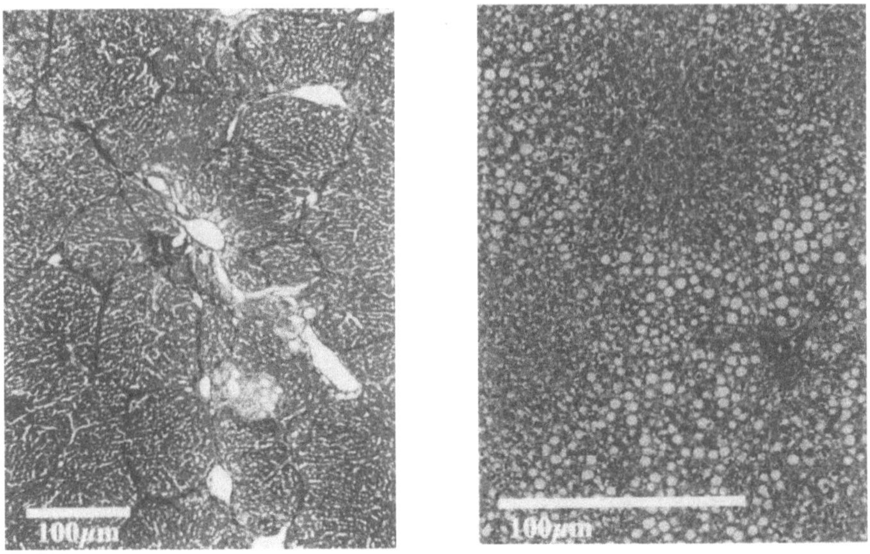

Fig. 4. (**a**) Livers of Wistar rats after chronic administration of carbon tetrachloride showing histological changes compatible with moderate liver cirrhosis. Slight to moderate periportal hepatic fibrosis was produced without nodules. (**b**) After a choline-deficient diet, livers of Lewis rats developed moderate steatosis; that is, fatty droplets were deposited in about 40–60% of hepatocytes

To determine if damaged livers also produce HSP72 after heat exposure and if livers pretreated by heat shock develop ischemic tolerance, similar protocols were tested on fibrotic livers (Shimabukuro et al. 1996) and steatotic livers (Yamagami et al. 1996). Fibrotic livers were produced by chronic administration of carbon tetrachloride (CCl_4) according to the method described by McLean et al. (1969) with some modifications. That is, the Wistar rats were allowed to access normal chow and sodium phenobarbital solution (0.5 g/l) freely. Two weeks after beginning the sodium phenobarbital regimen, subcutaneous injections of CCl_4 (0.2 ml/kg, diluted 1:4 in olive oil) were administered twice a week for the first 4 weeks and then once a week for the next 4 weeks. After these treatments, livers developed histological changes compatible with moderate liver cirrhosis (i.e., slight to moderate periportal hepatic fibrosis without nodules) (Fig. 4a). One week after stopping CCl_4 administration rats that had undergone heat shock preconditioning and those that had not were exposed to 30 min of warm ischemia.

Western blot analysis showed that the production of HSP72 was slightly stimulated just by chronic CCl_4 administration. On the other hand, the production of HSP72 was significantly stimulated in fibrotic livers 48 h after heat shock preconditioning. The 7-day survival after the 30-min warm ischemic load was only 21% in the group that had not undergone heat shock, whereas survival of the preconditioned group was 100%.

It seems that the vulnerability of the cirrhotic liver to warm ischemia occurs at a point similar to that of the protective effect of heat shock preconditioning. Because heat shock treatment did not influence morphological features of the fibrotic livers, this intervention seems to act within the molecular level of physiology. It is interesting to note that the serum transaminase levels were lower in the fibrotic livers after reperfusion in both the heat-shock and non-heat-shock groups than in those with normal livers; and there were no significant differences between the groups after reperfusion. The difference in transaminase levels between the groups became significant after 180 min with better values in the heat shock group. The precise reason for lower serum transaminase levels until 180 min after reperfusion in fibrotic livers is unknown. The formation of intervening basement membrane-like structures between the hepatic parenchyma and lumens of the vessels in fibrotic livers (Stenger 1966) may be responsible for a delayed release of transaminase from the destroyed hepatocytes.

Steatotic livers were produced in rats of the Lewis strain by feeding them a choline-deficient diet for 4 weeks according to the method described by (Hayashi et al. 1993). After these treatments, livers developed histological changes compatible with moderate liver steatosis; that is, fatty droplets were deposited in about 40–60% of hepatocytes (Fig. 4b). The production of HSP72 was obvious 48 h after heat shock preconditioning. In this experiment, warm ischemia was administered to the rats for 45 min because Lewis rats had been shown to be less vulnerable to ischemia–reperfusion injury in the preliminary study.

With this protocol the survival rate on postoperative day 7 was compared between the heat-shock-preconditioned group and non-heat-shock group, the survival rates being 87% and 33%, respectively, in the two groups. Energy status and serum transaminase levels after reperfusion were better maintained in the heat shock group and were similar to those in normal livers.

It has been reported that when a steatotic liver is exposed to warm ischemia severe liver failure develops, whereas a normal liver can tolerate the same period of ischemia without injury (Hui et al. 1994; Caraceni et al. 1995). In addition, it is well known that fatty liver grafts are difficult to preserve and easily fail after liver transplantation (Trevisani et al. 1996). Disturbances in microcirculation due to compressed sinusoidal spaces by fat droplets and swollen hepatocytes or the metabolic derangement of hepatic parenchymal cells are probable causes for the vulnerability of steatotic livers. Although at present we cannot define the precise mechanisms of heat shock preconditioning, severe congestion in hepatic sinusoids after reperfusion was strongly attenuated in the heat shock preconditioned steatotic livers. Because the obvious change in steatotic livers is the deposit of fatty droplets in hepatocytes, the production of reactive oxygen radicals during reperfusion is probably increased, and the succeeding pathologic signal pathways inside hepatocytes are stimulated by increased lipid peroxidation. Heat shock preconditioning and the overproduction of HSP72 may interfere with some cytoplasmic molecular cascades, suppressing the expression of adhesion molecules on sinusoidal surfaces. Further investigations in molecular biology should further clarify the mechanism underlying this phenomenon.

Ischemic Preconditioning

It has been reported that ischemic preconditioning of the heart or brain could result in the production of HSPs. We examined whether HSP72 is induced by means of ischemic preconditioning to the liver and if a tolerance to successive ischemia-reperfusion injury developed (Kume et al. 1996). Rat livers were preconditioned with short-term ischemia by cross-clamping the portal triad. Forty-eight hours after preconditioning, all rats were exposed to 30 min of warm ischemia and reperfusion. HSP72 was clearly produced in the liver 48 h after ischemic preconditioning, but not in the kidney or heart (Fig. 5). This experiment demonstrated that ischemic preconditioning also attenuated liver damage in the subsequent warm ischemia-reperfusion injury, improving the restoration of hepatic function during reperfusion and resulting in 100% postischemic survival.

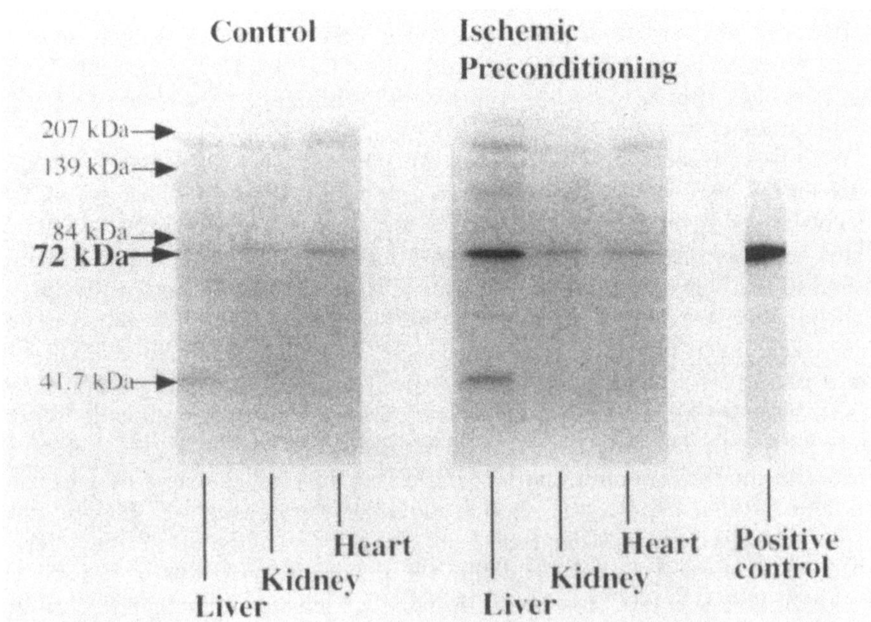

Fig. 5. HSP72 induction in the liver, kidney, and heart 48 h after ischemic preconditioning by portal triad clamping for 15 min. HSP72 was significantly produced in the liver 48 h after ischemic preconditioning but not in the kidney or heart. The protein concentrations are 9 μg/lane. The positive control is 0.2 μg/lane

Pharmacological Preconditioning

The possibility of initiating the stress response by pharmacological preconditioning was investigated using anticancer agents (unpublished data). Doxorubicin, *cis*-platinum, 5-fluorouracil, and mitomycin C were administered to rats by systemic intravenous infusion. Among these agents, only doxorubicin effectively induced the production of HSP72 in the liver. The induction of HSP72 by *cis*-platinum or mitomycin C was not as strong as that by doxorubicin. Administration of 5-fluorouracil failed to induce HSP72 in the liver. Doxorubicin exhibits its cytotoxicity by generating reactive oxygen radicals, which may effectively contribute to initiation of the stress response.

Doxorubicin was administered to rats of the Wister strain via the penile vein under anesthesia. At 48 h after administration, Western blot analysis demonstrated production of HSP72 in the liver. At 48 h after administration of doxorubicin, rats were exposed to 30 min of warm ischemia and reperfusion, and their tolerance to ischemia-reperfusion injury was examined. Survival on postoperative day 7 was more than 90% and was significantly better than the 50% demonstrated by the control group. At 40 min after reperfusion, biochemical parameters were also better in the doxorubin group. From these results, it can be speculated that doxorubicin can enhance the production of HSP72 and provide the liver with ischemic tolerance. Administration of doxorubicin prior to liver surgery therefore is expected to exhibit not only a neoadjuvant chemotherapeutic effect for cancer but also has the advantage of promoting ischemic tolerance in the liver during surgery.

Heat Shock Preconditioning for Chemical Injury

To represent chemical intoxication of the liver, the effect of heat shock preconditioning on CCl_4-induced acute liver injury was examined (Yamamoto et al. 1996). At 48 h after heat shock preconditioning, acute liver failure was achieved by administrating CCl_4 and mineral oil by gavage in all animals (Clawson 1989; Williams et al. 1990). Rats were sacrificed 24 h after the administration of CCl_4 and the serum transaminase levels, tissue adenosine triphosphate (ATP) levels, and histology of the liver tissue were examined. Transaminase levels were lower and tissue ATP levels were better maintained in the heat shock preconditioned group. Histological examination of liver tissue in the control group showed extensive necrosis of centrilobular cells and ballooning of hepatocytes located at the border of necrotic zones, whereas viable hepatocytes were well preserved in the livers of the heat shock preconditioned group. These results demonstrate that heat shock preconditioning apparently suppresses the poisonous effect of CCl_4. Although the usefulness of heat shock preconditioning in this process is still unknown, HSP72 may act to suppress free radical injury or facilitate the recovery of damaged hepatocytes by free radicals. Further investigation into its mechanism will facilitate the possible use of heat shock preconditioning to protect the liver during cancer chemotherapy.

HSP as a Stress Parameter

Because of the harmful effect of ischemia-reperfusion injury, investigation of the influence of portal congestion has been suggested (unpublished data). Currently it has not been clearly demonstrated. To determine the role of portal congestion in ischemia-reperfusion injury of the liver, liver damage after various combinations of hepatic ischemia and portal pooling was evaluated by measuring the accumulation of HSP72 in liver tissue.

Male Wistar rats were allocated to three groups. In *group P* the portal triad at the hepatic hilum was cross-clamped for 15 min to induce total hepatic ischemia with portal congestion. In *group S*, portal congestion was avoided by using an extracorporeal portasystemic shunt running from the coecal vein to the external jugular vein via a heparinized polyethylene tube. In *group C*, the superior mesenteric vein was occluded for 15 min to induce portal congestion without hepatic ischemia.

Biochemical parameters during reperfusion were suppressed better in group C than in the other two groups, and HSP72 was not detected in group C tissue. These findings suggest that in the absence of preexisting hepatic ischemia reperfusion of congested portal blood causes less damage. With respect to the reperfusion role of portal congestion associated with hepatic ischemia, biochemical parameters did not differentiate between the damage due to the reinflow of congested portal blood and that which incurred without the effect of congestion. These parameters primarily reflected ischemic damage of the liver. The production of HSP72, however, was remarkably higher in group P than in group S, illustrating the impact of congested portal blood on liver damage during reperfusion. In other words, the influence of portal blood congestion during reperfusion can be differentiated from other sources of ischemic liver damage by detecting the increased production of HSP72 in liver tissue.

The aspect of increased HSP72 production or overexpression of its messenger RNA in liver tissue may contribute to the assessment of liver damage, which is hardly detectable by conventional parameters. Moreover, because expression of HSP72 is an intracellular event, differences in the localization of HSP72 may be useful for evaluating the cytotoxic effect of chemotherapy, thereby differentiating a cancer lesion from a noncancerous area.

Future Aspects of HSP Study for Liver Cancer Therapy

Although the structures of HSPs have been well conserved throughout evolution and within species, their behavior in humans should be investigated separately. The important functions of HSPs are their regulation of the formation of tertiary structures in protein maturation by assisting the folding of newly synthesized proteins and the elimination of abnormal or denatured proteins. In cancer cells, where the cell cycle (and therefore, protein synthesis) are facilitated, it is relevant that specific HSP72 or HSC(HSP)73 is al-

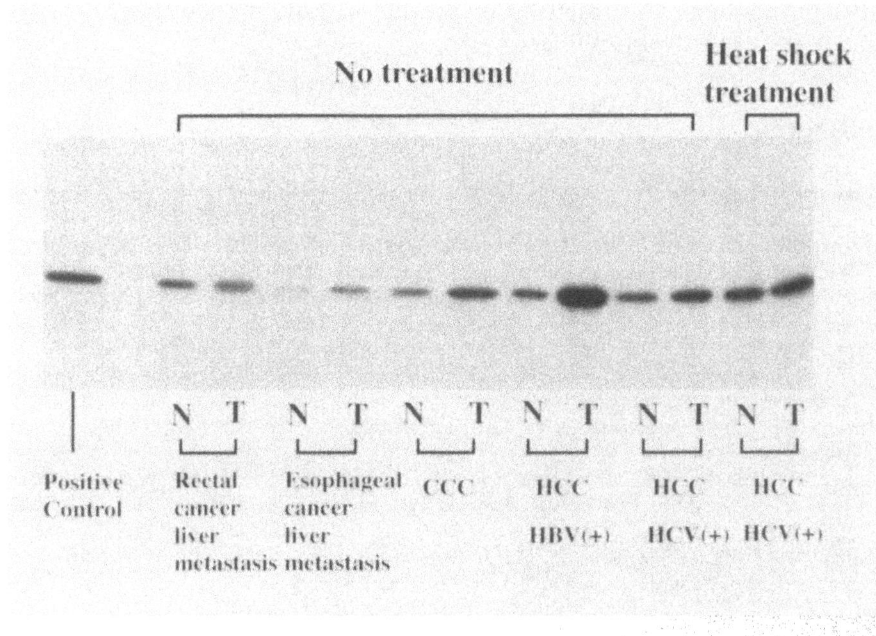

Fig. 6. Preliminary result of HSP72 expression in the human liver. Tumor tissues were obtained from primary liver tumors or liver metastases. Livers with viral infections produced more HSP72 than livers without infection. The production of HSP72 seemed to be stronger in tumor tissue than in nontumor tissues. In a heat-shock-treated patient, the production of HSP72 in the nontumor tissue was nearly the same as in tumor tissue. The protein concentrations are 3 μg/lane in specimens and 0.2 μg/lane in the positive control. *N*, nontumor liver tissue; *T*, tumor tissue; *HBV*, hepatitis B virus; *HCV*, hepatitis C virus

ready expressed without heat shock stress. In fact, some cancer cells are reported to produce HSPs without extrinsic stresses (Ferrarini et al. 1992). In our preliminary study, human liver tissue exhibited a low level of protein that reacted with mouse antibody against HeLa cell HSP72. The cholangiocellular carcinoma obtained from the same patient showed higher levels of HSP72 production (Fig. 6). It is worthwhile to determine if the synthesis of HSPs in cancer tissue due to heat shock stress is related to resistance to chemotherapy, and whether predicting the therapeutic effects of chemotherapy by analyzing HSP is possible. The comparison of HSP synthesis in cancer cells before and after hyperthermic perfusion chemotherapy in conjuction with its histological therapeutic effects has great potential for investigation. The degree of HSP production may depend on the type of liver cancer (e.g., hepatocellular carcinoma, cholangiocellular carcinoma, metastatic tumor) or on the degree of differentiation of the cancer. When noncancerous cells respond more sensitively to stress preconditioning, increased production of HSP72 will be ensured. Higher levels of HSP72 are expected to increase tolerance to the second stressor. This speculation corroborates the fact that repeated hyperthermia therapy has a more selective killing effect on cancer cells. In addition, the results may provide us with key information about tumor resistance to chemotherapy.

References

Ananthan J, Goldberg AL, Voellmy R (1986) Abnormal proteins serve as eukaryotic stress signals and trigger the activation of heat shock genes. Science 232:252–254

Bardwell JCA, Craig EA (1984) Major heat shock gene of *Drosophila* and the *Escherichia coli* heat inducible dnak gene are homologous. Proc Natl Acad Sci USA 81:848–852

Belghiti J, Noun R, Zante E, Ballet T, Sauvanet A (1996) Portal triad clamping or hepatic vascular exclusion for major liver resection: controlled study. Ann Surg 224:155–161

Caraceni P, Ryu HS, Gasbarrini A, Colantoni A, Demaria N, Trevisani F, Bernardi M, Van Thiel DH (1995) Alcohol-induced fatty infiltration increases anoxic injury in perfused rat hepatocytes (abstr). J Hepatol 23:154

Clawson GA (1989) Mechanisms of carbon tetrachloride hepatotoxicity. Pathol Immunopathol Res 8:104–112

Currie RW (1987) Effects of ischemia and perfusion temperature on the synthesis of stress induced (heat shock) proteins in isolated and perfused rat hearts. J Mol Cell Cardiol 19:795–808

Currie RW, Karmazyn M, Kloc M, Mailer K (1988) Heat shock response is associated with enhanced postischemic ventricular recovery. Circ Res 63:543–549

Ellis RJ (1990) The molecular chaperone concept. Semin Cell Biol 1:1–9

Ferrarini M, Heltai S, Zocchi MR, Rugarli C (1992) Unusual expression and localization of heat-shock proteins in human tumor cells. Int J Cancer 51:613–619

Finnell RH, Van Waes M, Bennett GD, Eberwine JH (1993) Lack of concordance between heat shock proteins and the development of tolerance to teratogen-induced neural tube defects. Dev Genet 14:137–147

Hahn GM, Li GC (1982) Thermotolerance and heat shock proteins in mammalian cells. Radiat Res 92:452–457

Hayashi M, Tokunaga Y, Fujita T, Tanaka K, Yamaoka Y, Ozawa K (1993) The effects of cold preservation on steatotic graft viability in rat liver transplantation. Transplantation 56:282–287

Heikkila JJ, Browder LW, Gedamu L, Nickells RW, Schultz GA (1986) Heat-shock gene expression in animal embryonic systems. Can J Genet Cytol 28:1093–1105

Hensler T, Köller M, Alouf JE, König W (1991) Bacterial toxins induce heat shock proteins in human neutrophils. Biochem Biophys Res Commun 179:872–879

Hightower LE (1980) Cultured animal cells exposed to amino acid analogues or puromycin rapidly synthesize several polypeptides. J Cell Physiol 102:407–424

Huguet C, Gavelli A, Chieco PA, Bona S, Harb J, Joseph JM, Jobard J, Gramaglia M, Lasserre M (1992) Liver ischemia for hepatic resection: where is the limit? Surgery 111:251–259

Hui A, Kawasaki S, Makuuchi M, Nakayama J, Ikegami T, Miyagawa J (1994) Liver injury following normothermic ischemia in steatotic rat liver. Hepatology 20:1287–1293

Hunt CR, Morimoto RI (1985) Conserved features of eukaryotic hsp70 genes revealed by comparison with the nucleotide sequence of human hsp70. Proc Natl Acad Sci USA 82:6455–6459

Kelly PM, Schlesinger MJ (1978) The effect of amino acid analogues and heat shock on gene expression in chicken embryo fibroblasts. Cell 15:1277–1286

Kume M, Yamamoto Y, Saad S, Gomi T, Kimoto S, Shimabukuro T, Yagi T, Nakagami M, Takada Y, Morimoto T, Yamaoka Y (1996) Ischemic preconditioning of the liver in rats: implications of heat shock protein induction to increase tolerance of ischemia-reperfusion injury. J Lab Clin Med 128:251–258

Landry J, Bernier D, Cretien P, Nicole LM, Tanguay RM, Marceau N (1982) Synthesis and degradation of heat shock proteins during development and decay of thermotolerance. Cancer Res 42:2457–2461

Levinson W, Opperman H, Lackson J (1980) Transition series metals and sulfhydryl reagents induce the synthesis of four proteins in eukaryotic cells. Biochim Biophys Acta 606:170–180

Li GC (1983) Induction of thermotolerance and enhanced heat shock protein synthesis in Chinese hamster fibroblasts by sodium arsenite and by ethanol. J Cell Physiol 115:116–122

Li GC, Meyer J, Mak YK, Hahn GM (1983) Heat-shock protection of mice against thermal death. Cancer Res 43:5758–5760

Lindquist S (1986) The heat shock response. Annu Rev Biochem 55:1151–1191

McAlister L, Finkelstein DB (1980) Alterations in translatable ribonucleic acid after heat shock of *Saccharomyces cerevisiae.* J Bacteriol 143:606–619

McLean EK, McLean AE, Sutton PM (1969) Instant cirrhosis: an improved method for producing cirrhosis of the liver in rats by simultaneous administration of carbon tetrachloride and phenobarbitone. Br J Exp Pathol 50:502–506

Morimoto RI, Sarge KD, Abravaya K (1992) Transcriptional regulation of heat shock genes: a paradigm for inducible genomic responses. J Biol Chem 267:21987–21990

Ohtsuki T, Matsumoto M, Kuwabara K, Suzuki K, Taniguchi N, Kamada T (1992) Influence of oxidative stress on induced tolerance to ischemia in gerbil hippocampal neurons. Brain Res 599:246–252

Parker CS, Topol J (1984) A *Drosophila* RNA polymerase II transcription factor binds to the regulatory site of an hsp 70 gene. Cell 37:273–283

Polla BS (1988) A role for heat shock proteins in inflammation? Immunol Today 9:134–137

Ritossa FM (1962) A new puffing pattern induced by a temperature shock and DNP in *Drosophila.* Experientia 18:571–573

Saad S, Kanai M, Awane M, Yamamoto Y, Morimoto T, Isselhard W, Minor T, Troidl H, Ozawa K, Yamaoka Y (1995) Protective effect of heat shock pretreatment with heat shock protein induction before hepatic warm ischemic injury caused by Pringle's maneuver. Surgery 118:510–516

Shimabukuro T, Yamamoto Y, Kume M, Kimoto S, Yamagami K, Yamamoto H, Ozaki N, Yamaoka Y (1996) New insight of protective strategy for the ischemia-reperfusion injury to the liver with fibrosis. In: Kim JP, Condon R (eds) Proceedings of the 15th World Congress of Collegium internationale Chirurgiae Digestivae. Monduzzi, Bologna, pp 341–344

Stenger RJ (1966) Hepatic sinusoids in carbon tetrachloride induced cirrhosis: an electron microscopic study. Arch Pathol 81:439–447

Thaddeus S, Nowak JR (1985) Synthesis of a stress protein following transient ischemia in the gerbil. J Neurochem 45:1635–1641

Tissieres A, Mitchell HK, Tracy UM (1974) Protein synthesis in salivary glands of *Drosophila melanogaster:* relation to chromosome puffs. J Mol Biol 84:389–398

Trevisani F, Colantoni A, Caraceni P, Van Thiel DH (1996) The use of donor fatty liver for liver transplantation: a challenge or a quagmire? J Hepatol 24:114–121

Velazquez JM, Lindquist S (1984) Hsp70: nuclear concentration during environmental stress and cytoplasmic storage during recovery. Cell 36:655–662

Welch WJ (1992) Mammalian stress response: cell physiology, structure/function of stress proteins, and implications for medicine and disease. Physiol Rev 72:1063–1081

Williams AT, Burk RF (1990) Carbon tetrachloride hepatotoxicity: an example of free radical-mediated injury. Semin Liver Dis 10:279–284

Yamagami K, Yamamoto Y, Kume M, Kimoto S, Yamamoto H, Okamoto R, Ozaki N, Yamaoka Y (1996) Protective effect of heat shock preconditioning on the warm ischemia-reperfusion injury in steatotic rat liver. In: Kim JP, Condon R (eds) Proceedings of the 15th World Congress of Collegium Internationale Chirurgiae Digestivae. Monduzzi, Bologna, pp 345–348

Yamamori T, Yura T (1982) Genetic control of heat-shock protein synthesis and its bearing on growth and thermal resistance in *Escherichia coli* K-12. Proc Natl Acad Sci USA 79:860–864

Yamamoto H, Kume M, Kimoto S, Shimabukuro T, Shigenaga H, Yamagami K, Yagi T, Yamamoto Y, Ozaki N, Yamaoka Y (1996) Protective effect of heat shock protein 72 on

CCl_4 induced acute liver injury. In: Kim JP, Condon R (eds) Proceedings of the 15th World Congress of Collegium Internationale Chirurgiae Digestivae. Monduzzi, Bologna, pp 353–356

Yellon DM, Pasini E, Cargoni A, Marber MS, Latchman DS, Ferrari R (1992) The protective role of heat shock stress in the ischemic and reperfused rabbit myocardium. J Mol Cell Cardiol 24:895–907

Xiao H, Lis JT (1988) Germline transformation used to define key features of heat-shock response elements. Science 239:1139–1142

Towards Gene Therapy for Colorectal Liver Metastases

M.M. van der Eb[1,2], R.C. Hoeben[2], and C.J.H. van de Velde[1]

[1] Department of Surgery, K6-R, Leiden University Hospital, PO Box 9600, NL-2300 RC Leiden, The Netherlands
[2] Laboratory of Molecular Carcinogenesis, Department of Molecular Cell Biology, Leiden University Medical Center, Wassenaarseweg 72, NL-2333 AL Leiden, The Netherlands

Abstract

Hepatic gene therapy may provide a new approach to treating hepatic malignancies. A promising strategy involves the infection of tumor and liver cells with replication-defective adenoviral vectors carrying suicide genes. The products of these genes convert prodrugs into cytotoxic derivates. In the transduced cells the subsequently administered prodrugs are thus activated and destroy replicating tumor cells, whereas the infected liver cells are thought to be unaffected because of their minimal proliferative activity. A major concern about this approach is that the suicide genes can theoretically enter the germline and other organs with high mitotic activity and as a consequence, cause their destruction. In vivo gene delivery should therefore be tissue-specific, and methods for targeted gene delivery are required. Targeting the colorectal liver metastases is pursued by combining the suicide gene principle and the surgical technique of isolated perfusion of the liver.

Introduction

The advancing technology of gene therapy has opened new avenues to the treatment of human disease. A prerequisite for gene therapy strategies to be effective and safe is to restrict expression of the foreign gene in the organs or tissues of interest. Cell- or tissue-specific targeting of the vector harboring recombinant DNA can be accomplished by (1): the route of administration of the vector; (2) the construction of vectors that specifically transduce predetermined cell types; and (3) tissue-specific expression of the transgene using tissue-specific promotors to drive the transgene. Many groups explore the latter two aspects. Modification of the fiber protein of the adenovirus, or the envelope protein of the retrovirus, may be used to modify the range of cell types that can be transduced. In addition to these studies, other targeting methods focus on the use of tumor-specific promotors, e.g., carcinoembryonic antigen (CEA) or α-fetoprotein (AFP) promotors (Vile 1994). Only in tumor cells that express these proteins can the promotor function, with initi-

Recent Results in Cancer Research, Vol. 147

ation of transcription of the gene-encoding sequences. Other theoretically promising targeting options are under investigation, but such discussion is beyond the scope of this paper.

More pragmatically, however, gene therapy clinical protocols have already been started employing the local delivery of recombinant DNA. For example, clinical trials using local delivery through bronchial instillation of the adenoviral vector encoding the *CFTR* gene for patients suffering from cystic fibrosis (Crystal et al. 1994). Isolated liver perfusion (ILP) might be another example of such a local delivery system that can be used for human gene therapy for liver diseases. Considering the complexity of this surgical procedure, ILP may be most useful for gene therapy protocols in which single administration of the virus is envisaged to suffice for a therapeutic effect, such as primary and metastatic cancer in the liver.

Suicide Gene Therapy

Among the various paradigms for cancer gene therapy, "suicide" gene treatment represents one of the most promising approaches. The best studied sui-

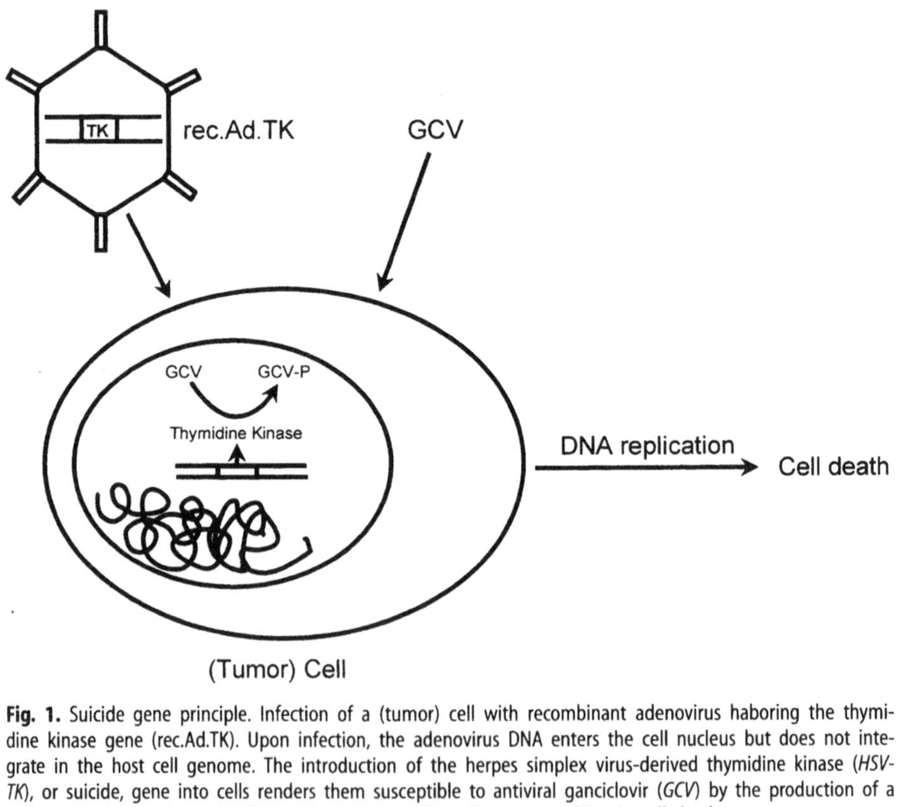

Fig. 1. Suicide gene principle. Infection of a (tumor) cell with recombinant adenovirus haboring the thymidine kinase gene (rec.Ad.TK). Upon infection, the adenovirus DNA enters the cell nucleus but does not integrate in the host cell genome. The introduction of the herpes simplex virus-derived thymidine kinase (*HSV-TK*), or suicide, gene into cells renders them susceptible to antiviral ganciclovir (*GCV*) by the production of a toxic nucleotide analogue (*GCV-P*) which inhibits DNA replication, resulting in cell death

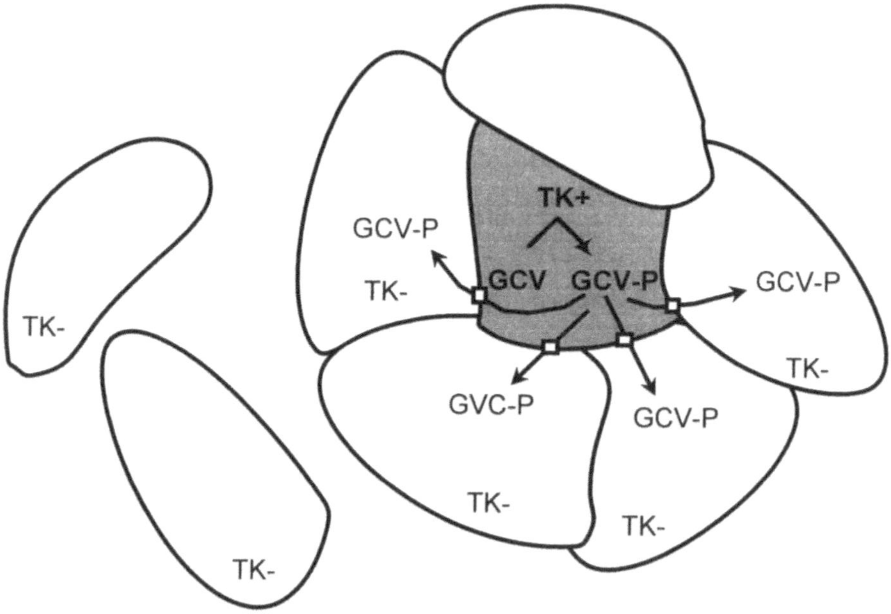

Fig. 2. Bystander effect. To achieve total tumor eradication, not all tumor cells need to express the HSV-TK gene. This phenomenon, known as the bystander effect, is attributed to the process of metabolic cooperation by which a toxic substance, phosphorylated ganciclovir (*GCV-P*), is transported between neighboring cells via gap junctions (□). Consequently, only those cells that are in direct cell-cell contact (TK-cells) with the thymidine kinase-transduced cells (*TK+*cells) receive GCV-P, whereas cells without direct cell contact *(TK–*cells) are not sensitized to this toxic compound

cide gene is the herpes simplex virus-derived thymidine kinase gene *(HSV-TK)*. Introduction of the HSV-TK gene into cells renders them susceptible to the antiviral drug ganciclovir (GCV) by producing a toxic nucleoside analogue that inhibits DNA replication (Culver et al. 1992; Caruso et al. 1993; Smythe et al. 1994; Qian et al. 1995) (Fig. 1). Rapidly dividing cells (e.g., tumor cells) have been shown to be effectively killed by such an approach, but cells that do not divide (e.g., hepatocytes) are thought not to be affected by exposure to ganciclovir (Moolten 1986). With this system, quantitative gene transfer is not essential as only a fraction of tumor cells must be *TK*-positive for complete tumor ablation to occur. It is due to the "bystander effect" (i.e., metabolic cooperation and transfer of activated toxins between neighboring cells) (Freeman et al. 1993; Chen et al. 1995; Colombo et al. 1995) (Fig. 2).

Vector systems

Introducing foreign genes into cells requires a vehicle for transportion. Three systems are widely used for this purpose: retrovirus-derived vector systems, adenovirus-derived vector systems, and non-virus-derived vector systems (e.g., liposome-protein-DNA complexes and naked DNA). Initially, retrovirus vectors were employed to transfer genes into cells, but because this approach requires target cells to be replicating only actively dividing cells can be transduced. This selectivity is advantageous for targeting rapidly dividing tumor cells, but gene transfer after either intratumoral injection of retrovirus vectors or implantation of irradiated vector virus-producing packaging cells has resulted in relatively low transduction efficiency (Naviaux and Verma 1992; Grossman et al. 1995; Nabel et al. 1994).

Low infection efficiency has also been found for nonvirus vector systems. More recently, vectors derived from human adenoviruses (types 2 and 5) have emerged as promising vehicles for gene transfer (Rosenfield et al. 1991; Quantin et al. 1992; Le Galle La Salle et al. 1993). High transduction efficiencies have been shown in vivo with these vectors, in both dividing and nondividing cells. In the experiments presented in this study we therefore use recombinant adenovirus vectors.

Materials and Methods

Cells and Cell Culture

All cells were maintained in high-glucose Dulbecco's modified Eagle's medium (DMEM) supplemented with 10% fetal calf serum at 37 °C in a humidified atmosphere with 5.2% CO_2. Cell culture media, reagents, and sera were purchased from Gibco Laboratories (Grand Island, NY, USA); culture plastics were purchased from Greiner (Nurtingen, Germany) or Falcon (Lelystad, The Netherlands). The CC531 cell line is a 1,2-dimethylhydrazine-induced, moderately differentiated adenocarcinoma of the colon, syngeneic with Wag/Rij rats (Thomas et al. 1993). SW837, LOVO, HT-29, and LS-180 are human adenocarcinomas derived from primary colorectal tumors.

Construction of Stably Transfected Cell Lines. Plasmids containing genes encoding firefly luciferase (pMoLuc) and thymidine kinase (pAdTK) were each cotransfected with a neomycin resistance gene (pRSVneo) into semiconfluent CC531 cells using the calcium phosphate transfection technique (Graham and Van der Eb 1973). Cells were then grown in G418-containing medium (400 μg/ml) to establish cell selection for the transfected cells. At 10 days after cotransfection colonies of 10–20 cells were picked for derivation of monoclonal cell lines. All stably transduced cell lines were constantly kept under selection pressure using G418 300 μg/ml in the culture medium. Growth kinetics of these stably transduced cell lines were similar to that of the CC531 nontransduced cells in vitro (data not shown).

Viruses and Virus Techniques

Construction of the recombinant adenovirus vector Ad.CMV.βGal and the Ad.CMV.Luc under the control of cytomegalovirus (CMV) enhancer/promoter have been reported before. Replication deficient E1-deleted adenovirus vectors containing the *HSV-TK* gene under either the CMV enhancer/promotor or the major late promotor (MLP) were described before and were a kind gift from B. Bout (TNO, Rijswijk, The Netherlands).

The recombinant virus was propagated on 911 cells (Fallaux et al. 1996) and purified by cesium chloride density centrifugation. Titers of the viral stocks were determined by plaque assay using 911 cells (Fallaux et al. 1996). Briefly, adenovirus stocks were serially diluted in 600 µl phosphate-buffered saline (PBS) and 2% horse serum (HS) and were then added to the near-confluent 911 cells in six-well plates. After a 30-min incubation at room temperature, the medium was replaced by F-15 minimal essential medium (MEM) containing 0.85% agarose (Sigma, St. Louis, MO, USA), 20 mM HEPES (pH 7.4), 12.3 mM $MgCl_2$, 0.0025% L-glutamine, and 2% HS. In vitro infections of all colorectal tumor cell lines were performed using adenovirus stocks diluted in 600 µl PBS/2% HS and added to 60–70% confluent six-well plates for 30 min at room temperature. Virus-containing dilutions were then removed and, after washing, replaced by culture medium.

β-Galactosidase Histochemistry. For detection of β-galactosidase activity, cells were fixed 48 h after infection in ice-cold 2% parafomaldehyde/0.2% glutaraldehyde solution, washed in ice-cold PBS containing 2 mM $MgCl_2$, and incubated in 5 ml of reaction mix [X-gal 1 mg/ml (Boehringer, Mannheim, Germany), 5 mM potassium ferrocyanide, 5 mM ferricyanide, 2 mM $MgCl_2$ in PBS] at 37 °C for 4–16 h.

Luciferase Assay. Cells that were exposed to Ad.CMV.Luc were lysed using cell culture lysis reagent (Promega, Madison, WI, USA). After a 15-min incubation at room temperature, the lysed cells were collected and briefly centrifuged to remove cell debries. The luciferase activity present in 20 µl lysate was determined by adding 100 µl of luciferase-assay reagent (Promega). After 10 s of preincubation the produced light was measured for 10 s in a luminometer (Lumat LB9501; Berthold, Wildbad, Germany).

Hepatic Metastases Model of Colon Carcinoma

Outbred male Wag/Rij rats (Harlan/CPB, Zeist, The Netherlands), weighing 200–250 g, were used for in vivo experiments. Cultured CC531 cells, syngeneic to Wag/Rij rats, were harvested by trypsination, and viable cells were counted and diluted in Hanks balanced salt solution to a concentration of 5×10^5 cells/50 µl and stored on ice until injection. For tumor cell implantation, a median laparatomy was performed and the major three liver lobes were located. About 5×10^5 cells were injected subcapsularly using a 0.45-gauge needle. Established tumors were measured with microcalipers on day 21. Tumor sizes were calculated by multiplying maximal tumor length and maximal tumor width. After removal, part of each organ was snap-frozen in liquid isobutanol and stored at -80 °C; the remainder was fixed in 3.7% formaldehyde.

Adenovirus Gene Transfer

For ex vivo gene transfer, cultured CC531 cells were infected with Ad.CMV.βGal and Ad.CMVTK at a multiplicity of infection (MOI) of 25, when 60–70% confluency was reached. Briefly, cells were incubated with virus stocks in PBS/2% HS for 30 min at room temperature. Cells were then washed, and medium was added to them. The cells were harvested the next day and prepared for subcapsular liver injection as described previously.

For in vivo gene transfer CC531 cells were implanted as described earlier. Six days after tumor cell injection the rats were reopened, the intestines were exteriorized, and the portal vein was located. Viral particle-containing buffer (1 ml) was slowly injected into the portal vein.

Results

Isolated Liver Perfusion for Liver-Specific Delivery of Adenoviruses

We have demonstrated that ILP can be used to achieve liver-specific transfer of recombinant adenovirus vectors (De Roos et al. 1997). In the experiments of De Roos et al. (1997) the adenovirus carrying the marker gene luciferase was used to compare the efficiencies of gene transfer to the liver and gene leakage to other organs after ILP and intraportal injection (IPI). A significantly higher gene transfer efficiency ($P = 0.028$) was found in the ILP group (mean 5.2×10^6 light units/mg protein) compared to that with IPI (mean 1.1×10^6). After IPI considerable luciferase activity could also be detected in most other organs (including kidneys, spleen, intestine, heart, lung, and gonads). Although low levels of luciferase activity could also be detected in some organs of a small number of animals after administration of the vector by ILP, the exposure to other organs was significantly reduced.

Adenovirus-Mediated Gene Transfer into Tumor Cells

We tested several human colorectal tumor cell lines (SW837, HT-29, LS180, LOVO) and one rat colorectal tumor cell line (CC531) for adenovirus-mediated gene transfer using Ad.CMV.βGal marker genes. Each cell line showed a high infection efficiency with Ad.CMV.βGal at MOIs of 30–100; there were up to 95% β-galactosidase-positive cells (not shown).

Tumor Cell Sensitivity to Suicide Gene Transfer and GCV Treatment

The CC531 cells were infected at MOI 0, 1, 2, 5, 10, and 25 with either Ad.MLP.TK or Ad.CMV.TK. They were subsequently grown in culture medium with or without ganciclovir (10 μg/ml). Although both the Ad.MLP.TK-infected cells and the Ad.CMV.TK-infected cells showed a clear sensitivity to GCV treatment, there was a significant difference in effect between the two adenovirus constructs. After 5 days of GVC treatment no viable cells were counted when infected with Ad.CMV.TK, whereas infection with Ad.MLP.TK and treatment for 8 days was barely sufficient to eradicate all tumor cells (Fig. 3).

In addition, human colorectal tumor cells were infected with Ad.CMV.TK at MOI 10 and treated with or without (controls) GCV. Viable cells were counted every 24 h using the trypan blue exclusion assay. All cell lines showed a significant inhibitory effect of the GCV treatment, whereas controls without GCV kept on dividing exponentially (data not shown). Two to three days after Ad.CMV.TK infection and GCV treatment, each cell line started to show abundant cell detachment, and cell viability decreased. One week after

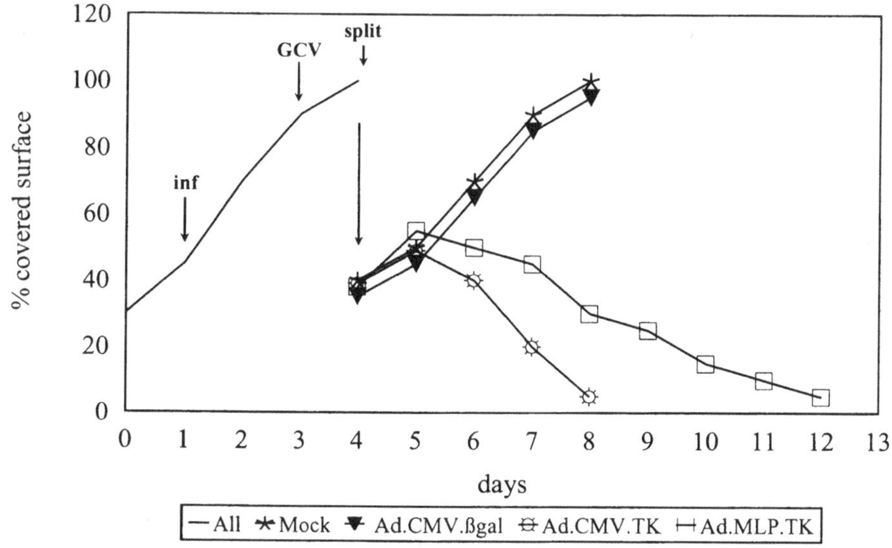

Fig. 3. Ganciclovir (GCV)-induced thymidine kinase-related cell inhibition of the CC531 cell line. CC531 were plated (day 0) and at 50–60% confluency infected with either Ad.CMV.TK (✲) or Ad.MLP.TK (□) at a multiplicity of infection (MOI) of 25 (day 1, *inf*). In parallel experiments, cells were infected with Ad.CMV.βgal (▼) or were mock (✳) infected as controls. At 48 h after infection GCV (10 μg/ml) was added to the culture medium (day 3). The covered surface was determined using Comassie blue staining of attached cells

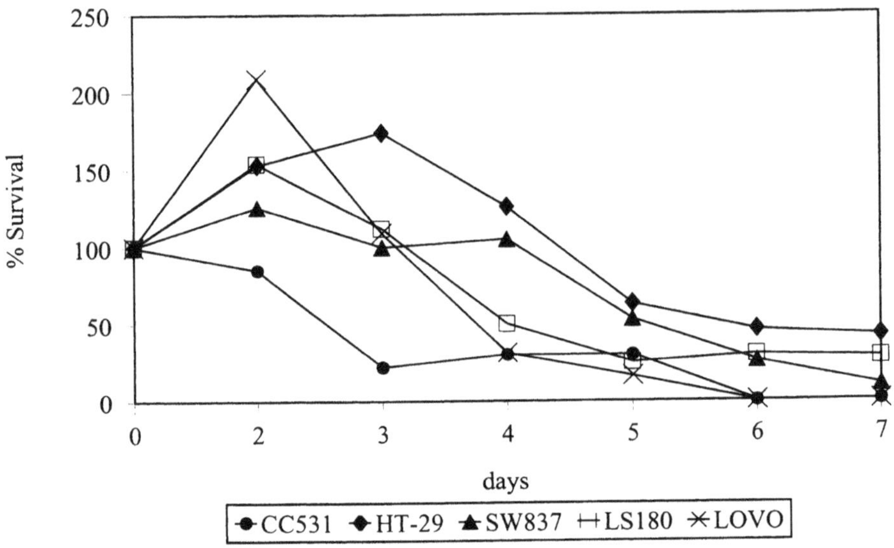

Fig. 4. Survival after Ad.CMV.TK infection and GCV treatment. After the cells were plated for 24 h, they were infected with Ad.CMV.TK at MOI 10. The next day GCV (10 µg/ml) was added to the culture medium. Every 24 h cell viability was determined by trypan blue exclusion. Controls without GCV grew exponentially (data not presented). *HT-29, SW837, LS180,* and *LOVO* are colorectal tumor cell lines derived from humans; the CC531 culture is derived from rat

initiation of the experiment the last cell count was performed; in the CC531, LOVO, and SW837 culture plates no viable cells were left, and HT-29 and LS-180 showed 70–75% cell inhibition (Fig. 4).

Potency of the Metabolic Bystander Effect to Kill Neighboring TK-Negative Cells

The ability of cells harboring the *HSV-TK* gene to kill adjacent cells was investigated using cell mixtures of stably transduced CC531 cell lines with pMoluc/pRSVneo and pAdTK/pRSVneo. Starting off with single-cell suspensions, cell lines were cultured at different ratios of CC531-TK/neo and CC531-Luc/neo: 0:1, 1:1, 1:2, 1:4, 1:8, 0:1, respectively in 3- or 10-cm dishes. Each experiment was set up in duplicate, allowing for one of the identical dishes to be cultured with GCV and the other without GCV, which provided an internal control for each mixture. Treatment with GCV was started when cells reached nearly 100% confluency to allow cell-cell contract to neighboring cells. After 2 days cells were transferred to larger cell culture dishes. Cell lysates were prepared 5 days after treatment, and luciferase activity was measured directly in equal amounts of the cell lysates. As only the pMoLuc/neo transfected cells express the luciferase reporter gene, and therefore extinct light, growth inhibition of these cells can be detected easily, comparing

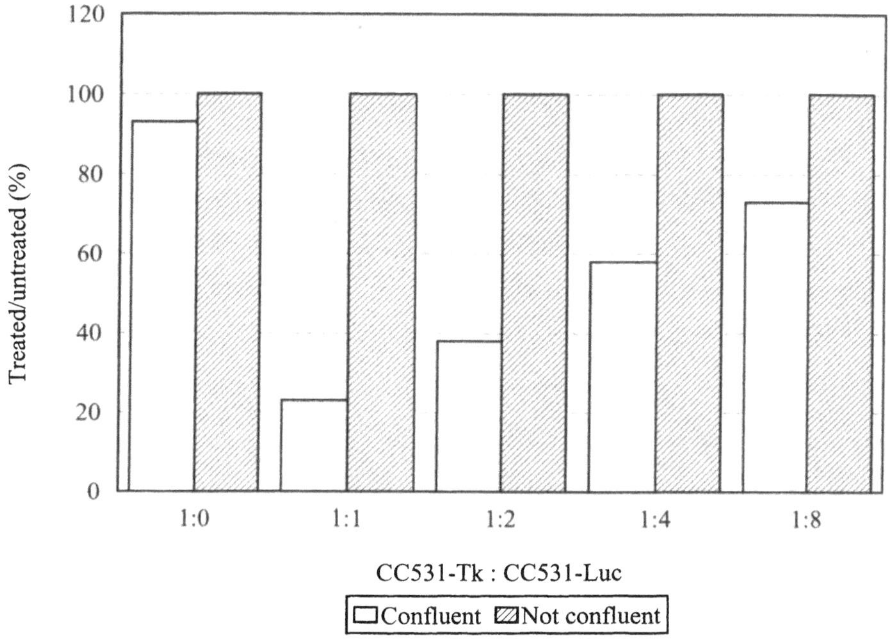

Fig. 5. Mixing experiments of stably transduced CC531 cell lines: CC531-TK/neo cells were mixed at various ratios with CC531-Luc/neo cells. Each experiment was performed in 3-cm dishes and 15-cm dishes to create a control without cell-cell contact. After reaching near-confluency in the small (3 cm) culture dishes, GCV (10 μg/ml) was added to the culture medium. Duplicate dishes served as controls and were not treated with GCV. Five days after treatment cell lysates were prepared, and luciferase activity was measured

treated cell lysates with the nontreated cell lysates. CC531-TK/neo cells only (1:0 mixture) showed no viable cells left, and obviously no luciferase extinction was measured. CC531-Luc/neo cells only (0:1 mixture) with GCV led to luciferase activity undistinguishable from that of the control without GCV. In cell mixtures with CC531-TK/neo and CC531-Luc/neo there was a significant decrease in luciferase activity in the duplicates with and without GCV. A greater share of CC531-TK/neo led to a greater difference; 50% of CC531-TK cells in the mixture allowed for a 67% decrease and 25% of CC531-TK cells resulted in a 42% decrease in luciferase activity compared to that in the internal control (Fig. 5). Although in the more diluted mixtures not all luciferase cells could be eradicated, these experiments clearly suggest a metabolic bystander effect.

Efficacy of Suicide Mechanism in CC531 Hepatic Metastases in the Rat

Having established the adequacy of the suicide gene approach for tumor cell kill in vitro we performed experiments to determine if it was also feasible in vivo. For this purpose CC531 colorectal tumor cells were infected in vitro with adenoviruses containing the thymidine kinase gene or *β*-galactosidase

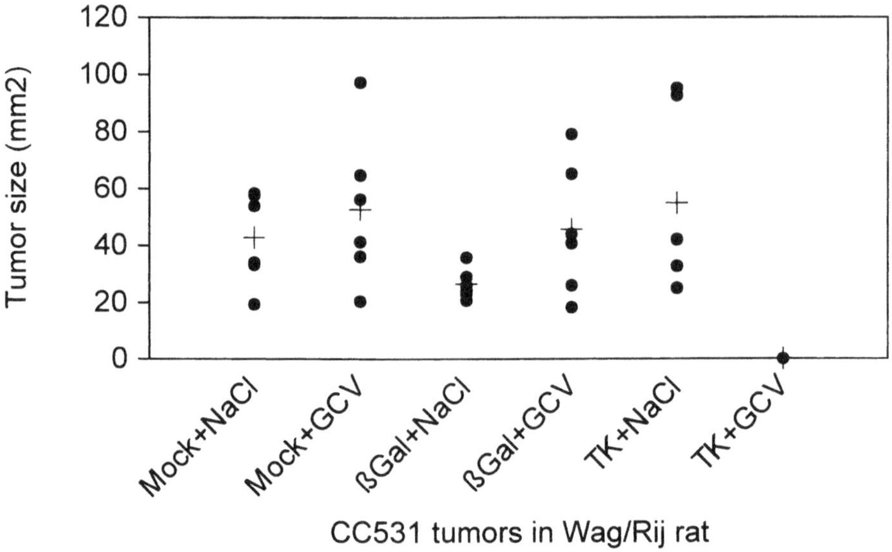

Fig. 6. Complete response of *TK*-positive tumors to GCV treatment in Wag/Rij rats. CC531 tumor cells were infected with Ad.CMV.TK ($n=12$) or Ad.CMV.βGal ($n=12$) or were mock-infected ($n=12$). After 14 h of culturing they were implanted in the liver. Half of each group ($n=6$) was treated for 18 days with GCV, and the other six were treated with saline. Tumor size was measured upon sacrifice at day 21. Each dot represents the mean tumor size per rat. The plus (+) represents the mean value of all rats in one group. Between-group differences were significant for *TK*/GVC compared to all other groups ($P<0.005$)

gene as control. Altogether 0.5 million tumor cells (CC531-TK, CC531-βGal, or noninfected CC531) were inoculated subcapsularly in the left, right and right accessory liver lobes of adult Wag/Rij rats. At 48 h after tumor cell infection, treatment was started with GCV ($n=6$) or saline ($n=6$) twice daily by intraperitoneal injection. Three weeks after tumor cell inoculation the rats were sacrificed and tumor size was measured using a microcaliper. Figure 6 shows the complete eradication of CC531-TK-expressing tumor cells after 18 days of GCV treatment. Control rats, inoculated with CC531-βGal or non-transduced CC531 cells, treated with GCV or saline, all showed reproducible tumor growth at the inoculation sites in the three liver lobes.

In Vivo Suicide Gene Transfer into CC531 Hepatic Metastases

Having provided the "proof of principle" in the above-described experiments, we studied the feasibility of in vivo gene transfer for treatment of colorectal liver metastases. For this purpuse, 5×10^5 CC531 tumor cells were inoculated subcapsularly in the left, right, and right accessory liver lobes of adult Wag/Rij rats. Six days after inoculation the tumors had each grown to 4–6 mm in diameter. To test the efficacy of adenovirus-mediated suicide gene transfer in vivo in these metastases, six rats were infused with 5×10^9 pfu

AdCMV.TK, 5×10^9 pfu Ad.CMV.βGal, or saline into the portal vein. At 48 h after infusion either ganciclovir or saline treatment was started (15 mg/kg per day IP twice daily). Three weeks after tumor cell inoculation the rats were sacrificed, and tumor size was measured. Tumors had formed in each of the control animals, although tumors were found in the TK/GCV-treated rats as well (not shown). Apparently the treatment with intraportally administered Ad.CMV.TK plus GCV hat not sufficed to induce tumor regression. Additionally, major liver pathology was observed in the Ad.CMV.TK and GCV-treated rats. Control rats showed no signs of this toxicity (M.M. van der Eb et al., in press).

Discussion

The liver is an important organ to target for gene therapy in patients with genetic disorders (e.g., hemophilia, familial hypercholesterolemia) and acquired disorders (e.g. hepatitis and cancer) (Chowdhury et al. 1991; Kay et al. 1993; Fallaux et al. 1995; Wilson 1996). In this respect, great potential lies in combining gene therapy protocols with ILP. Optimal gene therapy for monogenetic and polygenetic gene deficiencies or mutations require long-term expression from a dose of vector and repeated vector treatments. Considering the complexity of the ILP procedure, this route of administration will be most useful for gene therapy protocols in which single administration of the virus suffices for a therapeutic effect, such as primary and metastatic cancer in the liver.

Previously we demonstrated that ILP can be used to achieve liver-specific transfer of recombinant adenovirus vectors (de Roos et al. 1997). Additionally it was shown that the in vivo delivery of recombinant adenoviruses (rAdV) to the liver significantly reduces systemic leakage, the preventing unwanted exposure of nontarget tissues to the rAdV.

The present study demonstrates the feasibility of cancer gene therapy using suicide genes. Various colorectal tumor cell lines of rat and human origin could be effectively killed by Ad.CMV.TK and subsequent ganciclovir treatment. In the Wag/Rij rat model for colorectal liver metastases we established that transfer of the *TK* gene completely abolished tumor formation upon ganciclovir treatment. In the next series of experiments the vascular administration route of the adenovirus vector encoding thymidine kinase was evaluated by administration via the portal vein. Disappointingly, this strategy did not result in tumor regression. The reason may be that the virus dose used was insufficient. Another explanation may be the insufficient portal blood flow of established CC531 tumors 6 days after inoculation. In both cases ILP could overcome these problems. Unexpected, however, was the major toxicity found in the liver parenchymal tissue of Ad.CMV.TK- and GCV-treated rats. These preliminary data might imply limitations for the clinical application of the herpes simplex virus derived suicide gene. Further studies on the *HSV-TK* and GCV principle and the mechanisms of the observed toxicity must to clarify the possibilities for future application.

In addition to the TK/GCV suicide gene approach, other treatment strategies may be combined with ILP with respect to cancer gene therapy. Research currently is focusing on transfer of (1) other suicide genes that convert inactive prodrugs to cytotoxic compounds (2) genes encoding cytokines and stimulatory markers enhancing immune responses to solid tumors and (3) tumor-suppressor genes involved in the regulation of cell proliferation, apoptosis, and metastases.

1. In addition to the *TK* gene, other suicide genes have been developed, including the *Escherichia coli* cytosine deaminase gene (which renders tumor cells sensitive to the prodrug 5-fluorocytosine (5FC) by conversion to its active metabolite 5-FU) and the *E. coli* nitroreductase enzyme gene (which converts the weak monofunctional alkylating agent CB1954 to its highly active bifunctional metabolite) (Martin and Lemoine 1996).

2. Another promising approach envisages the use of gene transfer to elicit an immune response directed against the tumor cells. Controversially, the same immune reaction responsible for the failure of persistent expression of the transgene might be greatly beneficial in the generation of antitumor immunity and consequently long-lasting antitumor immunity.

A number of tumors express antigens that can be recognized by the immune system with the generation of specific cytotoxic T cells, but normal host immune responses are usually insufficient to cause tumor rejection. The potential induction of active antitumor immunity with gene therapy is therefore of particular interest. In this perspective several studies have shown that tumor cells transfected with genes encoding interleukin-2 (IL-2), IL-4, IL-6, IL-12, B7.1 interferon-α (INFα), or granulocyte/macrophage colony-stimulating factor (GM-CSF) are effective in reducing tumor progression and even curing established tumors in animal models (Galea-Lauri and Gäken 1996).

3. For many years research has been ongoing into the mechanisms of cell death. Opportunities are now opening up where this basic knowledge can be translated into new approaches to drug development for the treatment of various diseases. Gene therapy approaches using tumor-suppressor genes, such as *p53*, for the induction of apoptosis in (tumor) cells harboring a mutated form of *p53*, are now considered (Nielsen and Maneval 1998). Another interesting gene that has recently been cloned is the chicken anemia virus (CAV) *VP3* gene. In vitro expression of this single gene, also called *apoptin*, suffices to cause apoptosis in transformed cells. The fact that *apoptin* induces a *p53*-independent, *bcl-2*-insensitive type of apoptosis in human tumor cells and transformed cells, but not in normal cells, makes *apoptin* a potential antitumor agent (Danen-Van Oorschot et al. 1997).

Conclusion

Studies have shown the feasibility of applying ILP to liver-directed delivery of adenovirus vectors. Additionally, it was shown that recombinant adenoviruses are powerful vectors for the introduction of foreign genes into tumor cells. The nature of the above-described potential anticancer genes, together with the observed toxicity of normal tissues after thymidine kinase and GCV treatment in rats, emphasizes once more that for success of cancer-gene therapy the efficient and restricted delivery/expression of the therapeutic gene to the desired cell type is essential. Such tumor cell-specific gene expression can be achieved by a combination of localized gene delivery (i.e., via ILP), use of vectors with selectivity for dividing cells, and incorporation of specific transcriptional regulatory sequences to restrict gene expression to target cells.

References

Caruso M, Panis Y, Cangadeep S, Houssin D, Salzmann JL, Klatzmann D (1993) Regression of established macroscopic liver metastases after in situ transduction of a suicide gene. Proc Natl Acad Sci USA 90:7024–7028

Chen C, Chang Y, Ryan P, Linscott M, McGarrity CJ, Chiang YL (1995) Effect of herpes simplex virus thymidine kinase expression levels on ganciclovir-mediated cytotoxicity and the "bystander" effect. Hum Gene Ther 6:1467–1476

Chowdhury JR, Crossman M, Cupta S, Chowdury NR, Baker JR, Wilson JM (1991) Long-term improvement of hypercholesterolemia after in vivo gene therapy in LDLR-deficient rabbits. Science 254:1802

Colombo BM, Benedetti S, Ottolenghi S, Mora M, Pollo B, Poli C, Finocchiaro G (1995) The "bystander effect": association of U-87 cell death with ganciclovir-mediated apoptosis of nearby cells and lack of effect in athymic mice. Hum Gene Ther 6:763–772

Crystal RC, McElvaney NG, Rosenfield MA, Chu C, Mastrangeli A, Hay JG, Brody SL, Jaffe HA, Eisa NT, Danel C (1994) Administration of an adenovirus containing the human CFTR cDNA to the respiratory tract of individuals with cystic fibrosis. Nature [Genet] 8:42–51

Culver KW, Ram Z, Wallbridge S, Ishii II, Oldfield EH, Blaese RM (1992) In vivo gene transfer with retroviral vector-producer cells for treatment of experimental brain tumors. Science 256:1550–1552

Danen-Van Oorschot AA, Fischer DF, Grimbergen JM, Klein B, Zhuang S, Falkenburg JH, Backendorf C, Quax PH, Van der Eb AJ, Noteborn MH (1997) Apoptin induces apoptosis in human transformed and malignant cells but not in normal cells. Proc Natl Acad Sci USA 94:5843–5847

De Roos WK, Fallaux FJ, Marinelli AWKS, Lazaris–Karatzas A, Alting Von Geusau B, Van der Eb MM, Cramer SJ, Terpstra OT, Hoeben RC (1997) Isolated-organ perfusion for local gene delivery: efficient adenovirus-mediated gene transfer into the liver. Gene Ther 4:55–62

Fallaux FJ, Hoeben RC, Briet E (1995) State and prospects of gene therapy for the hemophilias. Thromb Haemost 74:263–273

Fallaux FJ, Kranenburg O, Cramer SJ, Houweling A, Van Ormondt H, Hoeben RC, Van der Eb AJ (1996) Characterization of 911: a new helper cell line for the titration and propagation of early region1-deleted adenoviral vectors. Hum Gen Ther 7:215–222

Freeman SM, Abboud CN, Whartenby KA, Packman CH, Koeplin DS, Moolten FL, Abraham GN (1993) The "bystander effect": tumor regression when a fraction of the tumor mass is genetically modified. Cancer Res 53:5274–5283

Galea-Lauri J, Gäken J (1996) Cancer Gene Therapy II: Immunomodulation strategies. In: Lemoine NR, Cooper DN (eds) Gene Therapy. BIOS Scientific publishers Ltd, Oxford, UK, pp 277–292

Graham FL, Van der Eb AJ (1973) A new technique for the assay of infectivity of human adenovirus 5 DNA. Virology 52:456–467

Crossman M, Raper SE, Kozarsky K, Stein EA, Engelhardt JF, Muller D, Lupien PJ, Wilson JM (1994) Successful ex vivo gene therapy directed to liver in a patient with familial hypercholesterolaemia. Nature [Genet] 6:335–341

Kay MA, Rothenberg S, Landen CN, Bellinger DA, Leland F, Toman C, Finegold M, Thompson AR, Read MS, Brinkhous KM (1993) In vivo gene therapy of hemophilia B: sustained partial correction in factor IX-deficient dogs. Science 262:117

Le Gal La Salle C, Robert JJ, Berrard S, Ridoux V, Stratford-Perricaudet LD, Perricaudet M, Mallet J (1993) An adenovirus vector for gene transfer into neurons and glia in the brain. Science 259:988–990

Martin LA, Lemoine NR (1996) Direct cell killing by suicide genes. Cancer Metastasis 15:301–316

Moolten FL (1986) Tumor chemosensitivity conferred by inserted herpes thymidine kinase genes: paradigm for a prospective cancer control strategy. Cancer Res 46:5276–5281

Nabel EG, Plautz GE, Nabel GJ (1994) Recombinant growth factor gene expression in vascular cells in vivo. Ann NY Acad Sci 714:247–252

Naviaux RK, Verma IM (1992) Retroviral vectors for persistant expression in vivo. Curr Opin Biotechnol 3:540–547

Nielsen LL, Maneval DC (1998) P53 tumor suppressor gene therapy for cancer. Cancer Gene Ther 5:52–63

Qian C, Bilbao R, Bruña O, Prieto J (1995) Induction of sensitivity to ganciclovir in human hepatocellular carcinoma cells by adenovirus-mediated gene transfer of herpes simplex virus thymidine kinase. Hepatology 22:118–123

Quantin B, Perricaudet LD, Tajbakhsh S, Mandel J-L (1992) Adenovirus as an expression vector in muscle cells in vivo. Proc Nat Acad Sci USA 89:2581–2584

Rosenfeld MA, Siegfried W, Yoshimura K, Yoneyama K, Fukayama M, Stier LE et al (1991) Adenovirus-mediated transfer of a recombinant α_1 antitrypsin gene to the lung epithelium in vivo. Science 252:431–434

Smythe WR, Hwang HC, Amin KM, Eck SL, Davidson BL, Wilson JM, Kaiser LR, Albeda SM (1994) Use of recombinant adenovirus to transfer the herpes simplex virus thymidine kinase (HSVtk) gene to thoracic neoplasms: an effective in vitro drug sensitization system. Cancer Res 54:2055–2059

Thomas C, Nijenhuis AM, Timens W, Kuppen PJ, Dalmen T, Scherphof GL (1993) Liver metastases model of colon cancer in the rat: immunohistochemical characterization. Invasion Metastasis 13:102–112

Van der Eb MM, Cramer SJ, Vergouwe Y, Schagen FHE, van Krieken JHJM, van der Eb AJ, Borel Rinkes IHM, van de Velde CJH, Hoeben RC (1998) Severe hepatic dysfunction after adenovirus-mediated transfer of the herpes simplex thymidine kinase gene and ganciclovir administration. Gene Therapy, in press

Vile RC (1994) Tumor-specific gene expression. Cancer Biol 5:429–436

Wilson JM (1996) Round two for liver gene therapy. Nat Genet 12:232–233

Subject Index

Springer and the environment

At Springer we firmly believe that an international science publisher has a special obligation to the environment, and our corporate policies consistently reflect this conviction.

We also expect our business partners – paper mills, printers, packaging manufacturers, etc. – to commit themselves to using materials and production processes that do not harm the environment. The paper in this book is made from low- or no-chlorine pulp and is acid free, in conformance with international standards for paper permanency.

SPRINGER NATURE

GPSR Compliance

The European Union's (EU) General Product Safety Regulation (GPSR) is a set of rules that requires consumer products to be safe and our obligations to ensure this.

If you have any concerns about our products, you can contact us on ProductSafety@springernature.com

In case Publisher is established outside the EU, the EU authorized representative is:

Springer Nature Customer Service Center GmbH
Europaplatz 3
69115 Heidelberg, Germany